REJUVENATION

REJUVENATION

or,

"My Birthday-Suit Doesn't Fit Me Any More!"

A Guide to
Nutrition, Exercise and Attitude

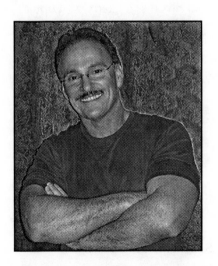

KEN COUNTS, PH.D.

BLUE DOLPHIN PUBLISHING

Published by Blue Dolphin Publishing, Inc.
P.O. Box 8, Nevada City, CA 95959
Orders: 1-800-643-0765
Web: www.bluedolphinpublishing.com

ISBN: 978-1-57733-157-5

Library of Congress Cataloging-in-Publication Data

Counts, Ken, 1949-
    Rejuvenation : or, my birthday-suit doesn't fit me any more!" : a
guide to nutrition, exercise and attitude / Ken Counts.
        p. cm.
    ISBN 978-1-57733-157-5 (pbk. : alk. paper)
    1. Nutrition—Popular works. 2. Exercise—Popular works. 3. Attitude
(Psychology) I. Title.

RA784.C62245 2007
613.7—dc22

                                                          2007009070

Cover art by Tito Salomoni, www.prestigeart.com
Used by permission.

Printed in the United States of America

10   9   8   7   6   5   4   3   2   1

Dedication

Dedicated to the loving memory of my parents,
Harold and Elfleeta Counts,
who both departed in 2005.

Contents

Foreword

THIS IS NOT ANOTHER DIET BOOK filled with false promises; in fact, it's not a diet book at all.

What you will read is the latest nutritional information from medical science translated by a professional who has spent years helping people cope with personal challenges.

This is a special combination. Most of us have a general idea of how we should lose weight and become more fit, and goodness knows, the bookstores are filled with information on nutrition and exercise. The problem, of course, is that adhering to a diet is not easy. That's where having the insight of an experienced, practical clinical psychologist comes in and makes this book a valuable resource.

As Dr. Counts points out, diets don't work. A large medical study that compared the traditional American Heart Association low-fat diet with the Atkins low-carbohydrate diet showed greater weight loss in the low-carbohydrates group at six months. But at one year, neither diet worked: both groups had gained back to their starting weights.

It's discouraging not just for cardiologists like myself who watch patients fail to keep their weight off or exercise regularly despite repeated urging, but, I suspect, for the reader and millions of others trying to improve their health.

Dr. Counts offers us some very helpful words that may well turn frustration into success. He points out that the ability to change one's self isn't just about a new diet or another resolution to exercise; it has a lot to do with one's emotional well-being and self-perception.

Understanding our own behavior, what makes us happy or otherwise, may well be the key to adopting a life of good choices in our diet and activity and successfully sticking with those choices.

Ken Counts is well qualified to help you understand this behavior. His remarkably successful practice as a clinical psychologist belies the fact that his approach to people with problems is practical, understandable, and, above all, works.

Ken shares his special knowledge about people and behavior in this book, coupled with a well-researched and readable review of modern nutrition and exercise science. What results is a powerful message that may redefine our medical approach to obesity in America; it will undoubtedly lead many readers to the same success in self-improvement that has been a hallmark of Dr. Counts' career.

Robert A. Lambert, MD, FACC
Cardiologist
Heart Clinic Arkansas

Acknowledgments

MANY PEOPLE HAVE BEEN INFLUENTIAL in the development of my life focus, including this text. I would like the opportunity to single out a few who have made a dramatic difference and some who provided direct support to this manuscript.

Dr. Bill Nutter, my collegiate track coach and physical education professor, demonstrated a scholar's approach to physical fitness that had a powerful, lasting impact on my thinking. He did not just talk the talk; he walked the walk. He served as a coach, a teacher and a mentor to me.

One of my under-graduate psychology professors, Dr. Bobby Williams, had a profound impact (I'm sure much more than he ever realized) on my education, achievement and professional development. Without his influence, my life was headed in another, very different direction.

My special thanks also to so many of the local physicians for their friendship and patience in teaching me many aspects of their profession. The medical community that surrounds me is exceptional and we all continue to learn together.

Thanks go out to all of my patients, from whom I continue to learn so much. They define my work and guide my continued education. They also warm my heart. I also extend much gratitude to my training partners for many years, especially Jon, Kevin, Peggy and others. We had a wonderful time.

My sister-in-law, April Counts, worked diligently in editing this manuscript, which was not an easy task. When she finished, I wasn't sure that English was my native language. Many thanks and much love.

My beautiful and wonderful daughters have always been inspiring, loving and supportive. The rest of my family and friends were terrific in their encouragement and reassurance.

Last, but not least, my beloved Tracey, for her tireless efforts to put together the rather extensive meal plans and recipes contained in this book. She developed them, cooked them, and we ate them. She did a fabulous job.

Introduction

MY REASONS FOR WRITING THIS BOOK ARE QUITE VARIED. Originally, it began with my writing various pieces of information as handouts for my patients. Over the years, these handouts began to accumulate into quite a bit of information. One day while I was rummaging through the various documents to give as handouts, a patient said, "Hey, Doc, you ought to write a book." Well, okay, I thought. I then began scanning through many books and papers and discovered what I thought was, at the least, misinformation if not just poor advice.

I had done much research on nutrition and how it relates to obesity and other health problems. Even though I am a psychologist, I have always tried to consider the "whole person." You see, many (if not most) of my patients also have other medical concerns and I try to be cognizant of those in regard to my treatment with them. Also, I have spent years studying exercise physiology and strength training because of my own personal hobbies. Exercise is something that I routinely recommend to my patients because of its many benefits. It is valuable as a stress outlet, and general conditioning seems to improve some emotional as well as medical conditions. Self-esteem is terribly important, and improved fitness and body image can often bolster self-esteem.

I also think that it is critically important to present my patients with various coping strategies to aid them in stress management and problem solving in general. I'm always looking for new ideas in this area. The purpose for having all of this information was to assist each of my patients in achieving a healthier lifestyle and a more positive personal psychology. For me, quality of life is the name of the game.

My other reason for accumulating so much information on nutrition is entirely personal. You see I had my own battle with health issues. That began about fourteen years ago when I finally acquiesced to having a routine physical. You know, blood work, lab work, chest X-ray, etc., just the usual stuff. I hadn't had a physical in many, many years. I knew it was not prudent to go that long without a physical exam, but I just didn't think it was necessary. After all, I thought, I had exercised religiously my entire life, and I saw myself basically as "strong as a bull." Well, the physical exam proved to be quite an eye opener and disconcerting. My cholesterol was sky high at 352; I discovered that I had high blood pressure and what appeared to be glucose problems. At that time I didn't know there was such a thing as glucose intolerance. Additionally, my doctor also weighed me and then asked, "How much weight have you gained?" I looked at the scale for a moment and I said, "Looks like about 30 pounds." I was amazed.

So there I was, early middle age and I know now that I had Syndrome X. Of course, I didn't know what that was then, either. So, I began taking my blood pressure medicine as prescribed and went on a low fat diet as my doctor had recommended. Yes, I really did cut the fat, but I continued to eat all of the carbohydrates that I wanted and did not pay any attention to what kind of carbohydrates. Well, fortunately my cholesterol did drop some to around 250 (still high) but my weight was still gradually going up. I was extremely frustrated about this. I also noticed that I had the tendency to have fairly high blood glucose after eating certain carbohydrates. I was concerned about this because Type II Diabetes runs in my gene pool.

At about this time I discovered the glycemic index in a book written for diabetics. That book was *The Good News Eating Plan for Type 2 Diabetics* by Elaine Magee. The concept of the glycemic index was new to me, but I found it very illuminating, and I quickly began to incorporate the concepts into my own diet. You know what? It worked! My weight began to drop—nice, predictably and slowly. My blood chemistry improved dramatically. Of course, I was still exercising, and that was a very helpful measure, too, and I am sure that it played a major role in my weight loss. By now, my cholesterol is actually normal, but I continue to be mindful of it.

In general, I don't think that diets work very well. I know that might seem like a surprising statement, but it's true. If they did, I don't think that we would have the rate of obesity that we do in this country. After all, we Americans are preoccupied with diets, and all that dieting does not appear to have had much impact on obesity in general. However, I have learned that changing my relationship with food helped dramatically. That is, changing lifestyles does work and can help with long-term weight loss. What I was doing was including a lot of healthy foods into my diet and excluding some unhealthy foods. You can be sure that I was still eating plenty and that what I was eating was very tasty. If it had not been satisfying, I probably would not have continued it. Since I liked what I ate, it was easy to stick with it and get healthier.

It was about that time that all of the low carb/no carb diets hit the bookstands with great popularity. I began to see people eating pounds of meat and cheese a day and I am thinking to myself, "I really don't think that is very good for you." You see, I have learned that many carbohydrates are really good for you and won't necessarily make you gain weight. I have also learned that fruits and vegetables are exceedingly healthy foods and it would be a danger and a shame to exclude them from our diets. I think it would probably shorten our life expectancy if we eliminated them.

As previously mentioned, exercise has been very good to me. It has allowed me the ability to continue virtually every activity I have ever enjoyed, and has certainly kept me young (at least inside my head and that's important, too). Body image can also have a powerful impact on self-esteem. I have always believed that exercise can help with the management of stress and even help treat depression as well as improve various medical problems. Exercise is a very important health-enhancing behavior— and this is true both medically and psychologically.

You see, my work is primarily concerned with people and their pursuit of their happiness. Control of stress is of course important in this regard. When I started seeing some research on the relationship between stress, obesity, health problems and mood disorders, I began to realize then that all of these issues are interconnected. Of course! I should have thought of it before. Our mind is our body in a very real way, and our body is our mind. Each affects the other. Physical fitness can pave the way for emotional fitness and vice versa.

This manuscript is not my attempt to write the quintessential diet or exercise book. It *is* my attempt to aid the reader in taking better care of themselves holistically—mind and body. There are many diet books (but diets don't work, remember). There are an almost unlimited number of fitness books, except people don't seem to be able to stick with those very long, either. Psychological factors are the missing link. They are the crucial variables in determining the outcome of nutrition, exercise, or any other personal growth endeavor.

This book is my attempt to demonstrate this interconnectedness between how we feel psychologically and how we feel physically. I have also attempted to provide practical information that can help the reader implement strategies that can really begin to transform their lives. I am encouraging changing health behaviors or lifestyle changes that can profoundly affect the quality of life, physically and emotionally.

The rejuvenation lifestyle is not a supporter of the "Peter Pan complex." It is not about avoiding growing up. Not at all. It is about enjoying life to the fullest, and I think looking and feeling young can be a great part of that. I also think it's terrific to be able to hang on to physical abilities for as much of your life-span as possible. I hate to see people "throw in the towel" on activities they have always loved. We all really need to play sometimes, and we need to be fit enough to play.

I fully understand that the acquisition of knowledge is a process and that science continually marches forward. That is, the scientific method is a process that illuminates new concepts and gives us new information. In my career I have seen this process predictably march forward with a plethora of new information obtained. Therefore, with all that said, I realize that some of the information in this book will likely be obsolete some day, and that some of my ideas will be replaced with new information and a better understanding. I am very content with that. Hopefully this current work will be helpful in the "stairway to knowledge" by at least providing one more step.

PART ONE

THE NEED
TO
REJUVENATE

CHAPTER 1

"What's Happening to My Body?"

GOOD GRIEF! Time flies, doesn't it? You still feel so young in your head, yet your body does not seem to reflect that. Our attitude may feel youthful, but our physical abilities just can't keep up. For most of us, there comes a time in our lives when we need to take a good, long look at ourselves and ask some solid questions about how we're taking care of the only body we will ever have. We also need to assess the quality of our lives and, perhaps, set some new goals or embark in a new direction. One of the keys here is to be brutally honest with the answers.

Does your "birthday suit" fit as good as it used to? Is it tighter in some places than it should be? Is it looser in some places than it should be? It could very likely be a bit of both. Ladies, are you carrying a little too much "junk in the trunk"? Yes, sometimes the "ole backside" (if you'll pardon me for being so bold) does broaden a bit. (What a shame!) Gentlemen, do you have any real need for that "spare tire"? Ah yes … the big belly. That's usually where we guys have a problem. And, where did your butt go? (I just know it's around here somewhere.) Father Time is so cruel. You may have hair growing out of your ears instead of on your head, but you can't keep your rear-end!

Do you remember what it was like when you occupied your skin well and how good that felt? Did you think that you could ever feel like that again? Or, do you see that as a distant memory which can only be recalled and not recaptured? I am here to tell you that you can go on farther than you can imagine in terms of recapturing that feeling. Also, do you remember when you were young and you could just "take off" and run across the yard effortlessly? When we were children, running was not work; it was play. Do you remember how good it felt to feel your body moving smoothly and fluidly? Do you also remember when you could jump and actually clear the ground? Wouldn't it be great to feel really good again? I'm here to tell you that you can! You'll be surprised at how far you can go. Don't you think it would be great to feel strong, firm and limber? I think most of us have had a moment when we thought, "What's happening to my body?" Wouldn't it be great to turn back your physiological clock? I sure think so! Wouldn't it be great to be *"rejuvenated"* and feel like you did five, ten, or more years ago? Would you believe me if I told you that, through your lifestyle, you could slow the aging process? Would you believe me if I told you that, in some cases, you could reverse it? Certainly, you can do this, but it does take some effort and some information. I want to provide you with the information and encourage you toward the effort. It's a life journey well worth taking.

LIFESTYLE

In my clinical practice, I have had the opportunity to observe many individuals. Some years ago, I began to notice that some individuals stay "younger" longer. It seems that some people seem to manage to maintain a more youthful and vital quality of life much longer than others. Perhaps you know someone who is forty-five or fifty years old that is still slim and trim and maintains a very active lifestyle. They probably look five to ten years younger than their actual chronological age. Maybe they play tennis or golf or other more vigorous sports and are able to enjoy a very active lifestyle. *Lifestyle* is the key word here. Essentially, we all reap the consequences of our chosen lifestyle. Poor diets can lead to nutritional problems, obesity, or both. Sedentary lifestyles can lead to premature loss of muscle mass and loss of health, loss of fitness, and, again, obesity. And smoking—well, we all know about smoking (don't get me started). Poor lifestyle choices catapult us toward premature aging, lack of fitness, disease, and even early death.

Several years ago I had the opportunity to go to the U.S. Master's Track and Field National Championship Track Meet. The Master's is a track and field competition for people over forty years of age. I was stunned and inspired by what I saw. I saw a group of people between the ages of forty and seventy-plus years old who were superbly conditioned athletes. The group of the younger participants (the forty to forty-five-year-olds) looked like collegiate athletes running around the track. These were strong, fast, energetic women and men who were having a ball playing as if they were eighteen years old. Many of them looked phenomenal for someone of any age. Emotionally, their attitude was "super-charged." They talked enthusiastically about their training regimes, their diets, and even their ability to overcome injuries. It was a terrific experience that renewed my commitment toward quality of life. You can find this lifestyle in other arenas, too. You can see people like this in gyms and health clubs across the country. You find them on tennis courts and sometimes golf courses. You find them at organized runs (such as 5k and 10k runs) and on the hiking trail, hiking up and down mountains. These people are participating in the activities that they love and are not giving up or in to the aging process.

On the other end of the spectrum, we probably also know individuals who are forty-five or fifty years of age who have multiple health problems, take multiple medications and appear to have incipiently begun to sink into old age. I don't think that's what any of us really want. I think that, too often, we get caught up in the immediate goals of day-to-day living, and we think we will plan a change soon. However, "soon" never comes. We just focus on getting through the day, and the days turn into weeks, the weeks turn into months, and the months turn into years. Before we know it, time has begun to pass us by, and we have hit the slippery slope that takes us to inactivity, health problems, poor body image and, often, low self-esteem. At this point, we often feel helpless or paralyzed. It seems that we have slipped so far that getting back is impossible. There's a kind of depression, or grief, that often sets in. The grief is from our perceived loss of previously enjoyed abilities. Also, there may be a change in our perception of our own physical body. If we look in the mirror or step on the scales and realize that we are 30, 40, 50, or more pounds overweight, it's very easy to feel overwhelmed and hopeless about the situation. Unfortunately, the depression can lead to inactivity which leads to increasing health problems, and we are then in a vicious cycle. Good attitude, or mood, is necessary for motivation, and motivation is necessary to change your lifestyle. It's all interconnected, but more about that later.

Not long ago a man came into my office who appeared to be sixty to sixty-five years old. I had not yet looked at his age on the paperwork in his new chart. As I began to talk to him, I was surprised to discover that he was only forty-seven years old. He was quite over-weight, and he had a diagnosis of diabetes as well as hypertension and chronic headaches. Unfortunately, this man had become a victim of his own lifestyle. He had been sedentary and had practiced poor dietary habits for most of his life. For the last five to ten years of his life, he had been overwhelmed with stress, leading to a state of rather chronic depression. This depression rendered him even more "paralyzed" than he was before. Depression often robs us of the energy and enthusiasm that we need to make positive changes in our lives. This man was caught up in that "vicious cycle" mentioned earlier. He felt so powerless that he found it very difficult to have any motivation to make a positive change. Sadly, he was no longer in any condition to enjoy some of the activities that he enjoyed when he was younger. Obviously, he did not have the endurance to play a game of tennis and probably would have difficulty walking more than a few blocks. I asked him a question that I often ask the people that I see. I asked, "What, in your life, are you looking forward to?" He could not give me an answer.

Folks, we desperately need to have things in our lives to look forward to. If we don't have them, then we need to create them. Regardless of where we are in our life's journey, we need to feel passionate about some things. This is part of how we realize meaning in our lives. Participating in life is *living*, and observing life is *only existing.* Activity spawns enthusiasm, and enthusiasm spawns activity, energy, and passion. I hope that the more you read, the more you will see this connection. The connection is that our physical health is, at least at times, related to our emotional health. The opposite can also be true. You see, happy and fulfilled people seem to have healthier lifestyles than people with depressed, anxious, or isolated lives. As a consequence, they often enjoy better health and fitness levels.

STRESS HURTS

Think, for a moment, how sad it is to allow the natural deterioration of our bodies to prevent us from enjoying life to the fullest. I began to look at some of the factors that affect our quality of life and noticed that diet and exercise were major factors in the ability to age well. In addition to this, psychological factors also appear to be quite important. Stress is a part of life for all of us, and it has the potential to be quite dangerous, so stress management is very important. We also definitely need a sense of purpose or meaning in our lives. This is vital in our quest for happiness. Developing a positive philosophy, or personal psychology, to aid us in our pilgrimage through life is as important as a roadmap is on a cross-country trip. We tend to get lost without it or, at least, head the wrong direction once in a while. Our personal psychology is our "guiding light" that helps us make decisions and increases our ability to constructively manage stress. It can aid us in our ability to develop outlets for stress and to achieve some degree of tranquility. Of course, we need to cultivate the ability to relax and find our peace.

Chronic, unresolved stress is correlated to obesity and other health problems. We're just beginning to understand this relationship and how important it may be in predicting positive outcomes from diet, exercise, or any other personal growth endeavor. I think it's so important that stress management needs to be a part of any diet plan. Also, a person's ability to manage stress and make important life decisions appears to be a critical factor in their quality of life, in general. Unresolved stress very often leads to depression, and depression produces a whole cluster of symptoms, including: poor sleeping (or sleeping too much), negative thinking, excessive guilt, low energy level, poor self-esteem, the inability to enjoy what used to be enjoyable activities, and concentration and memory problems. In short, depression can knock us "dead in the water." No question about it—this dreadful emotional condition can also be quite dangerous. It is a potentially deadly condition. Depression can rob us of the initiative to take good care of ourselves. As you can see from the symptoms of depression, it drains us of the ability to take self-enhancing steps in our life. It is exceedingly difficult, if not impossible, for a depressed person to engage in a high level of exercise or embark on a healthy nutritional plan. Therefore, learning to increase our tolerance of stress is a life skill that can have a profound effect on our wellness, and even that elusive quality that we all seek— *happiness.*

THE GOOD AND BAD OF GENETICS

With all that said, I understand the hard facts of genetics. They play a major role in health vs. disease as well as in our aging process. You can see evidence of this everywhere. There are families that are prone to obesity. There are families that are prone to being tall or lean. You even see elite athletes that produce offspring that become elite athletes (consider Archie Manning and his son Payton Manning, both exceptional athletes). We also know that many diseases have some genetic link. Heart disease, high blood pressure, and diabetes are just a few. For better or worse, our genetics do "hard wire" us toward certain conditions. They are so important that your doctor very likely has you fill out a family history before you first see him or her. This information is to discover what conditions or disorders you may be genetically prone toward. In many cases, the proneness to disease is just that—a proneness. It is not a guarantee that you will get the disease. Sometimes we can be genetically prone toward various disorders but are able to avoid them with our lifestyle. This is how potentially powerful our lifestyle choices are. These choices may empower us to avoid potentially life-threatening conditions. We may not get to choose our genetics, but that doesn't mean we have to view them as a "doomed to disaster" life. We should make every effort possible to avoid lifestyle choices that contribute to the disease or disorder. We each play a very powerful role in our own healthcare—*I think, the most powerful.* That's right, you're in charge! Whose life is it, anyway?

THE TIME IS NOW

Very often I see people in their forties, fifties, sixties or more that say "I used to..." and they complete the sentence by saying, "walk," "hike," "swim," "work out," "ski," "play softball," "bowl," "run," or some other activity. I think to myself, "That seems healthy and fun." Many times I ask them, "Why don't you do that now?" Most often the answer is some reference to age or health or both. Yet, I see other late-middle-aged people (I like that term, I guess, because I am one!) who are still at the gym, on the ball field, at the lake, walking the track, or engaging in other activities that are very healthy and enjoyable. In other words, they are participating in life. They are also *playing!* That's right. They are playing the game of life and having fun.

The time to get it together is now. Every day, week or month that goes by can be dealing out some real damage to your health if your diet is poor and your activity level is deficient. Like with so many things, the sooner you start the better off you are. The further down the fitness slope you go, the more difficult it will be and the longer it will take to recapture the benefits of rejuvenation. By the way, don't forget stress. The longer you live with unmanaged stress in your life, the more you risk obesity, disease, and emotional difficulties that can be quite severe. The time to act is now!

CHOICES

While genetic predispositions are certainly important, our choices also play a major role. Our choices regarding our lifestyle affect our health, fitness, and the overall quality of our life. When I use the term "lifestyle," what I mean is our dietary habits, our type and intensity of exercise, and our hobbies or leisure-time activities. It is also very important that we have skills or strategies we can use for tolerating and dealing with the stresses of life, as well as that successful philosophy of life or personal psychology.

Being a "baby-boomer" myself, I cannot help but notice how my particular generation has now become quite differentiated. In other words, some of us still seem to enjoy good quality of life in terms of physical abilities and the "happiness factor," while others appear to be at that place in life where they have begun to "throw in the towel" on their favorite activities and a general sense of well being. Some of us remain fairly disease free and others have a multitude of health problems. Obesity continues to increase, despite all we now know about nutrition, and concomitantly hypertension, diabetes, heart disease and other problems appear to be increasing health concerns. Some surveys suggest that these problems may indeed be epidemic in proportion, especially diabetes. Interestingly, it may be that lifestyle may play a large role in reducing the proneness to develop these particular disorders.

There have been a number of studies that indicate that diet and exercise habits play a very crucial role in avoiding these problems. Our lifestyle choices may indeed be helpful to us in terms of remaining healthy, and besides that, our lifestyle can be a deterrent to premature aging. I think that most of us want to look and feel as young as we can for as long as we can. Since there is no literal "fountain of youth," nutrition and exercise are probably the closest things to it. When you add a positive personal psychology, you have a winning combination.

I am going to challenge you and, hopefully, teach you how to reclaim some of the vitality of your youth. I am going to challenge you to slow down your own aging process. I want to teach you to "run and play" again. Let's get into condition and squeeze every drop of joy from our lives. I want each of us to have the very best quality of life that we possibly can. *Whose life is it, anyway?* Let's stubbornly refuse to "give up" on ourselves. I want us to put ourselves right in the middle of the equation of our life. Let's be a little selfish and refuse to participate in substandard nutrition and sub-par activity. I think we should adopt a positive philosophy or approach to life. Let's develop a self-enhancing personal psychology. Our fitness level can feed our positive emotions, and our positive emotions can feed our fitness level. After all, we are not divided into a mind and a body. In a very real way, *your body is your mind and your mind is your body.* Maximizing this inter-connectedness can maximize your life. The time is now to "wake up" and fully take charge of your life. Physically and emotionally the time to begin the change is now!

CHAPTER 2

Danger, Danger, Danger!

OBESITY

JUST A COUPLE OF GENERATIONS AGO, nutrition was poorly understood. Today, we are really beginning to understand nutrition and its effect on health. In spite of all our knowledge, however, obesity continues to be epidemic. Around 60% of Americans, age 20 or older, are considered overweight. A shocking one-quarter of our adult population is obese. From 1960 to 1994, the prevalence of obesity increased from 13.4% to over 22%. *That is a relative increase of more than 50%!* It appears that the prevalence of obesity increases with advancing age until around the age of 60; from that time on, it tends to decrease some. Of course, obesity is associated with a wide variety of medical problems, including heart problems, hypertension, diabetes and even cancer. **More than one hundred billion dollars is spent in the United States every year for care of chronic health problems that are often associated with obesity!** You see, this is no small problem. This is a huge and dangerous situation.

The future appears to look equally ominous. A recent study by the Center for Disease Control suggests that obesity will rival smoking as the number one cause of preventable death in our country. Can you imagine that? The key word here is "preventable." Can you believe that our overeating is rivaling smoking as a cause of death? No one questions the hazards of tobacco anymore. It is obvious that smoking represents an extreme insult to health and fitness. Now it appears that we are literally eating ourselves to death! It seems that poor diet and physical inactivity have caused 400,000 deaths in the year 2000. This is a 33% jump over 1990. Tobacco related deaths over the same period climbed by less than 9% to 435,000. As you can see, the gap between the two has narrowed considerably. At this rate, obesity will soon claim the top spot for death by preventable causes in the U.S. Again, pay attention to that word "preventable." The obesity problem can be changed but currently is a serious situation. You see, obesity is not a laughing matter at all. It is not only a threat to health and fitness; it is also a matter of life and death.

The prevalence of obesity is especially remarkable when you consider how much we now know about nutrition. It would seem that weight problems should be drastically decreasing. However, the opposite is true. Part of the problem is dieting. **You see, diets don't work!** Does that surprise you? Nope, there's precious little evidence that diets are effective in long-term weight management. If they were, I don't think we would be seeing the problems with obesity that we have in our culture. Yet, almost any diet can result in short-term weight loss, which means absolutely nothing in terms of consistency or stability of weight over time. That initial weight loss is mostly water, not body fat, but it gets people excited—at least for a while. Dieting in our culture has a "faddish" quality to it. People flock to this diet or that diet, singing the praises that finally someone has discovered the answer to the problem of weight. Then, the diets consistently fail. Think about the history of diets in the last twenty years or so. See what I mean? How many different diets have been presented in that time? Don't you think if there were a secret to weight control, it would have been discovered by now? And with all those diets, we are still not losing weight. No, in the strictest sense, diets don't seem to work. Again—just look at our country. What country diets the most? This country. What country is the fattest? Ditto! The good ol' U.S.A.

The problem that exists between dieting and weight loss is complex, and I would direct you to *Breaking the Rules of Aging* by Dr. David Lipschitz for further explanation. Dr. David's excellent work should be read in entirety, but in the first chapter he provides much information about why diets fail. One of the problems is that most diets represent a rather drastic change in the way a person normally eats and is a dramatic departure from the way he or she likes to eat. Therefore, people can stay on the diet for a while and then, inevitably, they will fail and with this failure comes the return of the weight, usually with a few extra pounds to spare. This yo-yo weight cycling is very hazardous to health and fitness regardless of age and condition. The dangers come in terms of blood chemistry problems, high blood pressure, and loss of muscle mass. None of this is good. The loss of muscle mass, alone, can slow the rate of metabolism and have a deleterious effect on future weight control. It is imperative to stop weight cycling. I think that weight cycling is more dangerous to your health than simply being overweight.

It appears there may be another really deceptive problem with dieting. The stress of dieting alone may trigger stress hormones that contribute to cravings and thus, weight gain. Amazing. Dieting creates a craving for calorie-dense foods. Well isn't that swell? Because dieting represents a change in our life (and is a stressor by definition) it may, in fact, support weight cycling. Okay then, what do we do? I think we have to add more healthy food to our diet while removing, at least some, high calorie or unhealthy food from it. I think this is the only way to lose weight and keep it off. Yes, it requires a change in lifestyle.

Let me give you an example. I once had a young male patient who was about thirty pounds overweight. He was having a terrible time trying to lose the weight. I finally said, "Why don't you try eating at least three small fruits a day and stop the soft drinks and see what happens?" He acknowledged that he did like apples, so I encouraged him to eat three small- to medium-sized apples a day. I encouraged him to do this by eating one in the morning, one in the afternoon, and one in the evening. Guess what happened? Well, he lost weight. Because he had added some healthy, nutritious food to his diet, he didn't experience as much hunger. That is, he felt full. Therefore, he ate a little less in terms of his normal daily diet. The apples took up some of his normal daily volume of food. Also considering the fact that he dropped some empty or junk calories naturally, he lost weight the right way. Yes, there is a right way to lose weight. While most diets are either too restrictive or represent too great of a change, long-term weight loss is still possible. Considering the dangers of obesity, there are some good reasons to lose weight as well.

SYNDROME "X"

In the last ten years or so, scientists have been making interesting discoveries regarding a condition that tends to precede disease. Have you heard of Syndrome "X" yet? This condition is sometimes called Insulin Resistance, Metabolic Syndrome or, occasionally, Carbohydrate Sensitivity. Let's look at what a syndrome is and is not. A syndrome is a group of symptoms that tend to occur or cluster together. That is, a syndrome is not considered a disease itself, per se, but this syndrome does suggest the likelihood of developing some significant diseases. Metabolic Syndrome X can be dangerous.

WHAT ARE THE SYMPTOMS?

The symptoms that cluster together to form Syndrome X are the following:

1) Central Obesity (that's a big belly, folks)—this is fat that tends to locate around the torso of the body, sometimes referred to as visceral fat.
2) Insulin Resistance, or Glucose Intolerance—I'll discuss this condition in more detail a little later, but it's basically the inability to get glucose into the cells of the body and out of the bloodstream.
3) Blood Fat Disorders—mainly, this is high triglycerides and low HDL cholesterol (that's the good cholesterol). This is also referred to as Atherogenic Dyslipidemia.
4) Raised Blood Pressure—that is a blood pressure elevated above 130/85 mmhg.
5) Pro-Inflammatory State—that means an elevated C-reactive protein in the blood indicating that you have an increased risk

of suffering a heart attack or stroke. This may have more implications than just high cholesterol alone. More and more, it appears that arterial inflammation is a potential killer.

6) Prothrombotic State—this is high fibrinogen in the blood. This appears to raise the probability of abnormal clotting. It is this clotting that can increase the incidence of heart attack or stroke.

As you can see and appreciate, Syndrome X is not just an inconvenience. It's very dangerous.

Insulin Resistance

Let's take a look at glucose intolerance or insulin resistance. So, what is insulin resistance? Insulin is a hormone that is secreted by the pancreas, which is a gland in the body. As carbohydrate is digested, it causes an elevation in blood glucose or blood sugar, which triggers the release of insulin from the pancreas; this insulin gets energy from the blood sugar and distributes it into our cells. That is, insulin takes the blood glucose (which is the body's fuel) and puts it into the cells where it can work and provide energy for the body. When people are insulin resistant, it means that their cells respond very sluggishly, or slowly, to the action of the insulin: the energy does not get into the cell, where it needs to be, and the sugar in the blood does not drop. Therefore, following a meal, this person will have elevated blood sugar circulating for some time. This produces high blood sugar, or high glucose levels, which can result in a predisposition to diabetes. To increase this rather sad state of affairs, if the blood sugar is too high, for a variety of reasons, it can increase the over-all appetite and, concomitantly, weight. And, to make matters even worse, the increased body fat may make the individual more insulin resistant, and so on. So, in effect, the problem "snowballs" and the situation can become more and more difficult.

As mentioned earlier, insulin resistant individuals generally have high triglycerides. Unfortunately, high triglycerides usually coincide with low HDL cholesterol. (We really need this good cholesterol). These blood lipid problems can have serious consequences over time, possibly leading to heart attack or stroke.

Remember, prevention is unimaginably more advantageous than treatment of these disorders. Improving blood chemistry is always important in terms of prevention and should certainly be considered in any and all diet plans. Changes in diet plans or nutritional planning should not just be about weight loss. Any nutritional change should be about improved health status.

At this time, there is no cause and effect relationship clearly established for this syndrome. I feel sure that excess body fat is a contributing factor, and that future research will give us a better understanding of the causes and effects of this condition. However, there is certainly reason for considerable concern regarding Syndrome X especially, since any of these symptoms alone, or in combination, can certainly increase one's risk for coronary artery disease or stroke. This is not an issue of fitness; it's an issue of life and death.

INCIDENCE

So, how many of you out there have this Syndrome X? Estimates of people with Syndrome X range from 10 to 25 percent of the adult population. The condition is more highly concentrated in individuals over 40 years of age. Yes, this is what my parents referred to as "middle age spread." Some estimates state that over the age of 50, one out of three individuals has Syndrome X. That is a lot of people. There is some evidence that it may be slightly more common in men than in women. As mentioned earlier, we men tend to carry excess body fat at the waist. Certainly, obesity is a major factor in the metabolic Syndrome X. So, how do we establish the severity of obesity? We are all familiar with those height/weight tables seen at the doctor's offices in the past. Personally, I don't think those were very useful. The newest notion is the body mass index (BMI). While this is an improvement, this is still basically a type of height/weight comparison and is somewhat limited. Perhaps it's okay to use with a completely sedentary population, but for individuals who exercise and have considerably more lean body mass, the BMI is just inaccurate. Some people simply look at waist size and consider a waist size of over 40 inches in men and over 35 inches in women as being obese. This is probably better than nothing, but it still doesn't take into consideration other physical variables. I think the best measure of obesity would simply be to obtain a body composition analysis, or measure the percentage of body fat and percentage of lean tissue. This can be done with the old skin fold measurements or some of the other newer techniques. Obtaining the percentage of body fat is not available to everyone and probably won't be, so I doubt that will set the standard; but it is the most meaningful measure. You might try checking with a fitness center or exercise physiologist. He or she should be able to check your body composition. A radiology group in my community has a program where they use a bone density scanner to determine body composition with extreme accuracy. Quite a few fitness enthusiasts are using this technique regularly to plot their progress. Body composition is assessing the percentage of the body weight that is lean tissue, the percentage of the body weight that is body fat, and even determining bone mass. It is also fairly economical; so, hopefully, services like this may become more common.

THE TREATMENT

Now for some good news: if you have metabolic Syndrome X, you can reverse it. If you don't have Syndrome X, you can avoid it. Changes in lifestyle can accomplish this, but the things that you have to do are more easily said than done. Certainly, you should monitor your blood sugar levels and your cholesterol. Also, you should keep track of your blood pressure, and if weight is a problem, you will have to lose some weight. Depending on your weight, it may be recommended that you lose 10 to 15 percent of your current body weight. Again, that is easier said than done, as I'm sure you well know. If you weigh 200 lbs., that is 20 to 30 lbs. of weight loss. We do know that weight loss can lower your blood pressure and increase your body's cell's sensitivity to insulin. That's a good thing! Weight loss can also have a therapeutic effect on your cholesterol levels. Of course, losing weight can be great for elevating your mood and dramatically improve your energy level.

Exercise is also an important component of treating Syndrome X. Not only is it an important component in weight loss, it also tends to raise HDL cholesterol blood levels. In fact, if you exercise, you may increase your HDL cholesterol levels *even if you don't lose weight* (that's always good!). Also, diet can help reduce triglycerides. Diets low in alcohol and simple, or high glycemic index carbohydrates (I'll talk more about this later), tend to reduce triglyceride levels. This does not mean a low carbohydrate diet. There are wide varieties of "good" carbohydrates that you can consume that have a therapeutic effect on your triglyceride levels. In fact, some fruits, grains, beans, and vegetables may help reduce triglyceride levels. With high triglycerides, and weight control in general, the total number of calories consumed a day should be considered.

In summary, Syndrome X, Metabolic Syndrome, or Insulin Resistance, or whatever you want to call it, is a potentially dangerous precondition for disease. Adequate steps can be taken to improve your chances of not getting the syndrome or to reverse the syndrome if you already have it. Good nutrition goes a long way toward reducing your symptoms of Syndrome X. While I'm going to cover nutrition more comprehensively in the chapters that follow, diet alone only goes so far. Exercise is a critical component in reducing the likelihood of developing serious problems from this Syndrome. Exercise is also crucial for enhancing health and fitness, and improving the quality and quantity of life. Incidentally, when it comes to exercise, I'm not a big believer in the conventional wisdom that walking the dog for twenty minutes, or taking the stairs occasionally, is the answer. I think that exercise should be *hard*. To have real health benefits from exercise, we must learn to push ourselves. Taking exercise seriously is the only way to enjoy the health benefits from it. I'll talk more about a comprehensive exercise program later because it is extremely important.

The treatment of Syndrome X should also involve some form of stress management. As mentioned earlier, obesity is often correlated with poorly managed stress. This relationship is both simple and complex. From the most basic standpoint, stress is a state of unease or discomfort, and eating "comfort" foods is something we can do right away to make us feel instantly better. Unfortunately, later we may feel guilty and otherwise disappointed with ourselves, and that only serves to increase our emotional stress. The whole process tends to repeat itself. Ah, another self-defeating cycle. Biologically it is much more complex.

Stress not only produces an array of psychological symptoms, it also produces a variety of physical changes. Of particular interest are the stress hormones. Both acute and chronic stress produce significant elevations in what I will term "stress hormones." These include adrenaline, noradrenalin and glucocorticoids, to name a few. These hormones seem to directly or indirectly influence body fat in general, and abdominal fat in particular. They can be viewed as playing a role in producing a "craving" from a biological standpoint due to their impact on the brain. These chemical changes may, in fact, trigger the urge to eat carbohydrates and especially sugar. Energy metabolism is also affected in such a way as to increase the probability of central obesity. At any rate, psychological coping strategies are extremely important in the treatment of Syndrome X.

I'm sure future research will illuminate many of the issues that we see in Syndrome X. However, for now, I think it is very important to get "little around the middle" through sound nutrition and scientifically based exercise. And yes, certainly, genetics play a role. Be extra wary if you have diabetes in your family. If you do have Metabolic Syndrome X, and your physician advises, there are medications available that can help, as well. If your lipids are out of control, I certainly recommend that you talk to your physician regarding the cholesterol lowering drugs that are available. The "statin" drugs are probably under-prescribed. The statin drugs appear to be generally safe, and they appear to have a very low side-effect profile. It also looks as though they offer additional health benefits that go beyond simply the reduction of cholesterol. These drugs may very well protect you from arterial inflammation, which is also a major player in the coronary artery disease game. Better safe than sorry. You don't want to play "coronary roulette." If you have some risk factors for heart disease, ask your physician about these options. Remember, you are in charge of your health care, so take that role seriously. Your doctor knows that you are the main variable in the equation of your health. So feel free to ask questions, share concerns, or give feedback to your health professionals.

CHAPTER 3

The Building Blocks
of Rejuvenation

NUTRITION

Now it's time to discuss nutrition—or diet. I know, it's the dreaded "D" word but it's not what you think. I am not talking "diet," like "I'm on a diet." I'm talking "diet"—like the way that you eat every day, all the time, forever. Remember, the word *diet* means "the foods normally consumed." Basically, you are on a diet now. The food you are normally consuming in the course of your days and weeks *is* your diet. This may not be particularly good, but it is still your diet. Too many times we think of diet as a predetermined amount of time that we endure unusual and undesirable food products; then, after we've suffered enough, we resume our normal dietary habits. Too often that's what a diet is, and that's one reason why they fail. That's when we get into the problematic weight cycling that was discussed earlier. Remember, this is not only counterproductive in terms of weight loss; it's also hazardous to your health. It is very important to avoid weight cycling. I would invite you to think of this nutrition plan as simply adding more nutritious, healthy, delicious food to your daily caloric intake and removing some specific food items that are clearly not good for you—that is, substituting sound nutrition items in place of calories from nutritionally void foods. As mentioned before, including some healthy food items will take up some "space" in your normal dietary volume. Dropping some unhealthy food items also contributes to this space.

Did you ever stop and ponder a question like this: "What are we supposed to eat?" That is, what should the human animal eat for optimum health? Another way of looking at it would be, "What are the natural foods for human consumption?" Surely, in the great scheme of things, there are foods that we are supposed to eat.

Although I have occasionally been called "the fitness doctor," I am neither a dietician nor a nutritionist, but a psychologist with a special interest in promoting healthy life styles, fitness levels, and enhanced quality of life. Therefore, with the aid of a great deal of fairly current research, I will address weight control and eating habits, or "eating behavior," which is probably a better way of putting it. How we eat is almost as important as what we eat, and I have some suggestions for eating behavior that are presented later. When discussing nutrition, we must always give some thought to the macronutrients. This seems to be the arena where all the dieting "fuss" abounds.

The role of proteins, carbohydrates and fats seems to remain a controversial topic and the controversy about these macronutrients will probably continue long after this writing. Fortunately, the science of nutrition will continue to provide new information that can be incorporated into practice as time marches on. Nonetheless, I will try to explain in a very simple way how your body utilizes the macronutrients. They are all important.

Proteins are, indeed, the building blocks of life. They are necessary for the maintenance and repair of our cells. Can you burn protein for fuel? Can you eat too much protein? We'll see.

Carbohydrates are what your body recognizes most readily as fuel. They are absolutely necessary for good health. While there is some confusion regarding carbohydrates, I will try to illustrate the vast differences that various carbohydrates have on your body. While some carbohydrates provide long-lived, high endurance energy for you, other carbohydrates provide a very quick burst of blood sugar that is so extensive that you are more than likely not going to be able to burn it up or utilize it as energy. Your pancreas has to work very hard to secrete a relatively large amount of insulin and when the blood glucose does drop, it plummets. Our brain detects this rapid drop in blood glucose. There seem to be many things that stimulate hunger, but one of those things is the rapid drop of blood glucose. Dropping glucose seems to hit a trigger point in our brain that stimulates hunger again. Of course, this hunger will stimulate the consumption of more calories which can lead to gaining more and more weight over time. This is not a good thing.

Have you heard of the Glycemic Index (GI)?—in general, it's the speed at which a carbohydrate is converted into circulating blood sugar or glucose: that is, how fast a carbohydrate will give up its sugar to the blood stream and be available for the cells. This seems to be a critical factor in how carbohydrates affect us, because high glycemic carbohydrates produce rapid rises in blood sugar (with the problems noted above) and low glycemic carbohydrates produce slow and low elevations in blood sugar. Generally, low glycemic carbohydrates will not make you fat and will fuel your body very well. These are very good carbohydrates. Not only do they provide good nutrition and necessary energy, they also seem to offer a feeling of fullness or satiety that prevents us from quickly feeling hungry again.

Dietary fats, too, can be graded in terms of positive or negative impact on your health and weight control. Some fats are absolutely necessary for optimum health and physical functioning. Not only is some fat good for you, we actually require these fats in our diets in order to avoid illness. Some fats may reduce LDL (bad) cholesterol and elevate the HDL (good) cholesterol. These "good" fats also may aid in a feeling of "fullness." However, some of the fats that are consumed are "married" to high cholesterol food sources. Certainly, we should severely limit the intake of fatty cuts of beef, pork, and the like. Cholesterol is still potentially dangerous and should not be taken lightly. Therefore, we should opt for the leaner cuts when we eat red meat and still not eat these too frequently. When it comes to fish, I actually recommend it without any regard to the frequency or the amount. Obviously, I would not recommend it being fried. Grilled or baked is fine. Chicken and turkey are protein sources and are excellent as long as you generally avoid the darker meat and the skin. You'd be surprised how much cholesterol can be there. Remember this is important in any nutrition plan because high cholesterol is still a major player in coronary artery disease.

EXERCISE

Physical exercise appears to be absolutely critical in the maintenance of a good quality life. Yes, you can lose weight through diet alone. This is also true of my nutritional plan. However, I think it is virtually impossible to reclaim the vitality of your youth without fairly rigorous exercise. Reshaping your body and adding lean muscle mass cannot be accomplished through diet alone. Diet should be viewed as necessary, but not sufficient. In order to reshape your body, you need to acquire some muscle mass while losing body fat, and that means employing a combination of diet and exercise. This change in body composition is an important element in the rejuvenation lifestyle. If you will, consider the body of the average 20-year-old person as compared to the average 40-year-old person. What do you think? I think you can see that decreased body fat and increased muscle mass is desirable and "youthing," not to mention the self-esteem aspects. A changing body contributes to a changing body image. Improved body image has an impact on self-confidence and feelings of security. Obviously, this impacts our self-esteem. Diet and exercise are both important and optimize each other.

We have a popular health food market in my community. I was there picking up some items the other day and stopped and sat on a bench outside for a few minutes. The business is quite successful and a large number of people were coming and going with items. As I "people-watched," I couldn't help but notice that quite a few of them were somewhat overweight. Others were thinner but still looked "flabby." I remember thinking to myself, "Sound nutrition is a great start, but it's only a start." Many of these individuals had clearly focused on their diet and took it very seriously, but they were still not enjoying optimum fitness. Doing your shopping at a health food market is a good start, but don't stop there! Exercise is a must.

Our human bodies have not changed much for many millennia. However, our diet and our activity levels have changed dramatically. The human body was obviously designed by God to prosper from hard work. Exercise contributes to biological efficiency and the human body adapts or adjusts to the physical stress placed on it. What this means is that the more you do, the more you will be able to do. What a beautiful biological reality! Conversely, the less you do, the less you are able to do. (I know, sad but true.) From the remote past, through the intermediate past, human existence was comprised of a great deal of physical activity. From the early hunters and gatherers that lived a no-madic lifestyle, through the Agricultural Era, humans worked hard. I'm sure, by modern standards, obesity was quite scarce. Life was difficult and filled with sometimes-grueling work. Like I said, the human body was designed by God to work and work hard.

Today, we have scientific and systematic ways of engaging in activity for health purposes. We've learned a great deal in the last century about how to most profit from exercise for health and fitness. Exercise physiology has yielded a tremendous amount of information, and continues to engage in research to further our knowledge. We know that we can exercise in the wrong way. We also know that we can, in fact, exercise too much. We have learned that different types of exercise yield different kinds of benefits. This knowledge allows us to develop an exercise model that yields maximum benefits for the body as a whole. It also allows our exercise to be very efficient. By exercising intelligently, we can get maximum benefits from a minimum investment of time—al-though, I should mention once again, the exercise should be hard. This means that the intensity has to be sufficient to produce these maximum benefits. One thing is for sure, regardless of our current level of functioning, we all need some form of exercise.

For practical purposes I am going to divide exercise into three main categories—Aerobic Training, Strength Training and Flex-ibility Training. Aerobic training, or cardiovascular conditioning, has proven beneficial for the cardiac and respiratory systems. It's fat burning by nature and probably can increase longevity, at least to some extent. It certainly can improve cholesterol levels, reduce blood pressure, and help manage stress. It also, of course, im-proves endurance. All that sounds good, and it's easy to see how this activity can enhance life.

Flexibility exercises are beneficial for the joints and connective tissues. It can also aid tremendously in stress management. Like so many other abilities, flexibility tends to decrease with age. Of course, that does not have to be the case. Like most of our abilities, flexibility decreases as a consequence of disuse. There are a variety of ways that stretching can be applied to any exercise program which will result in benefits gained.

Thirdly, strength training, or resistance training, has proven to be beneficial in maintaining muscle mass and strength and is also beneficial as a metabolic aid. Strength training has been found to improve bone density. You see, weight-bearing activities improve the strength of our skeleton. In addition to this, strength training can have a strong impact, psychologically, on our self-esteem and feelings of general well being. Find someone who lifts weights, ask them about it, and see what they say. They'll tell you it's great.

It is by combining these three modalities that you maximize your ability to enjoy life. Increased endurance and lower body fat, enhanced flexibility and increased muscle strength, that's the combination that sets the pace for "youthing" not "aging." What could be better?—looking younger, feeling younger and increased abilities to move—now we're talking *quality of life*.

STRESS MANAGEMENT

As you can see, virtually all forms of exercise are useful in stress management. Exercise becomes one of the many potential "outlets" for stress that we can develop in our lifetime. These outlets are critical for maintaining equilibrium in our lives. When we have greater incoming stressors than we have outgoing outlets, we are thrown into a state of distress that has varying, yet significant negative consequences. These negative consequences can be physical in the form of headaches, irritable bowel syndrome, ulcer disease, hypertension, or others. They can also be psychological in nature and produce anxiety and/or depression. Too often, unresolved stress produces both physical and emotional difficulties.

Also, I consider "stress management" as the enhanced ability to adjust to change. That's a general statement, understood, but the process of living exposes us to ever-changing realities. Our ability to successfully adjust to these changes increases our likelihood of not sustaining any damage from stress. It is also critical to develop an "emotional support network"—that is, relationships with others who nurture us, aid us in living, and, in general, make us feel loved and cared for. This is very important. Successful development of this emotional support system is vital to stress management and overall happiness. Dr. Dean Ornish's book, *Love and Survival*, is an excellent work depicting the importance of relationships and interconnectedness in our lives. Our connection with others not only enhances our happiness, but it also seems to improve our ability to recover from illness and injury. Dr. Ornish quotes numerous research projects that have demonstrated that our emotional wellness contributes significantly to our physical wellness. We are social creatures. Isolation tends to produce a depressive lifestyle and increases our chance for many diseases and disorders. Just as our bodies were designed for work, so are we fashioned for community and, indeed, we need love.

In fact, a regular exercise regime and healthy relationships with others will go a long way in terms of personal stress management. Note: "a long way," not all the way. It is also important, as we go through life, to be on the lookout for activities that enhance a sense of meaning or purpose in life. Activities that give us a sense of meaning become important outlets for stress, and they are also helpful in terms of our personal identity and self-esteem. It is extremely important to continue to search for activities that we feel passionate about and which are healthy for us, and to look to increase the "menu" of activities that we can enjoy in life. This search is an ongoing process.

Sound nutrition, intelligent exercise, and a positive personal psychology with stress management strategies, these are the building blocks of rejuvenation. They pave the way for an active, positive life and promote not just fitness but also health and happiness. Each of these building blocks is critical in terms of being able to fully enjoy your life. Isn't that what life is all about?

PART TWO

SOUND NUTRITION

CHAPTER 4

The Human Body—
What Should I Feed It?

OUR HUMAN BODIES have remained, in many ways, unchanged for many millennia. However, it is unbelievable how much our diets have changed over time. Let's ponder for a moment what the human animal should eat. There will be a wide degree of variation here. You see, we must first learn what is *"food"* and what is *"not food."* This knowledge is not innately present in our awareness. We learn it through a variety of channels. This is most often influenced by cultural and individual family expectations, as well as locale. For example, in some parts of the world, as you wean from mother's milk, you might be given raw fish to eat. If so, you would identify that as *"food."* Likewise, in other cultures, once you're weaned, you'd be given cereal to eat. Again, you would identify that as *"food."* If you were raised in a vegetarian culture, you would identify some plant sources as "food" but animal sources as "not-food." As you can see, there are many possibilities, and a great variation exists in different groups around the world. So we as individuals don't necessarily pick what we consider *"food"* or *"not-food."* Our culture, our parents, and our locale are highly influential in terms of what we identify as *"food."*

In our Western culture, for instance, let's say you are a baby being weaned and someone gives you a piece of a jelly donut. Because it is loaded with sugar and tastes good, you would most probably readily identify that as *"food,"* even though, of course, it is not. (What?! You say a jelly donut is not food?!). With all these possible variations, how do we identify what is, in fact, *"proper food"*? What is the natural diet for a healthy human? Even though huge differences occur around the world, some generalizations can be made about what is food and what is not food.

A BRIEF HISTORY OF FOOD

So what are we supposed to eat? What is the natural diet for humanity? To discover the natural diet of animals, biologists very often observe those animals in their normal, natural habitat. This way they can record what that animal eats of its own volition. In a similar vein it might be helpful if we could observe mankind in its natural habitat. This would be hard to do in our culture because there's not much left that would represent a natural habitat. (I don't think a recliner, a TV, and a remote count as natural habitat!) This might best be done historically, so let's go back to the late Paleolithic period, about 30,000–10,000 B.C. This seems like a good era to begin to identify items that make up the human diet.

Humans were the up-and-coming species, and anthropologists have been able to provide us with a surprising amount of information about the life of Paleolithic man. Let's designate a particular individual from that period and follow his behavior. We'll give our Paleolithic guy a name—let's call him "Bob." Bob is a member of a group, or clan, of human hunters and gatherers. That is, these early humans foraged for their entire diet. There were no gardens and no domesticated animals, so it is very likely that sometimes food choices were highly variable and at other times, the sources were quite restricted. For example, the changing seasons would have a huge impact on available food. Colder weather would suggest that more food was obtained from animal sources and, conversely, warmer weather would offer more plant foods.

Bob's food pyramid was actually not a pyramid at all but more like a block—a food block. You see, Bob's two main food groups were animal and plant, just as we have today. These plants and animals were part of his natural world and what was "food" may have been determined primarily by trial and error. This seems like a pretty tough way to identify food! Can you imagine the daring and bravery necessary to be the first person to eat, say, a crab? It is tasty to eat, but it doesn't look tasty to eat! I bet a lot of items were tried that were, indeed, quite nasty.

Now, Bob ate a huge amount of meat, and I do mean a lot, depending on what was available. Just about anything that crept, crawled, flew or swam was fair game, and he didn't waste much of it. He ate a lot of muscle tissue of the animals as well as the organ meat, including the liver, kidneys, brains and the like because these are very rich in nutrients. Bob even went further than that. He ate the marrow right out of the bones. He would crack the bones open with a sharp stone and eat the fatty, buttery marrow with relish because this too provided much needed nutrition. Paleolithic Bob would need to eat whatever he could, whenever he could, in order to survive. These fatty meats provided tremendous amounts of much needed energy. Bob never knew when he was going to be able to eat again. There could be, potentially, long periods of time from one meal to the next. It was important that he consume large quantities of meat, including the fat, for energy. He would eat all he could and carry away or store what he could not because that was necessary for survival. You can see that this same mentality has survived to the present era when you observe human behavior at an all-you-can-eat buffet. The problem is that Bob's eating instincts helped him to survive in his day, but that same tendency serves us quite poorly today. It seems our brain is still telling us to eat all we can, whenever we can. You can quickly see the difficulty this poses for us. For most of us, food is readily available almost everywhere. This is very different from our ancestors.

With Bob's scarcity of agricultural skills, he would have had an extremely difficult time getting enough nutrition from the plants because they are generally less calorie dense than animal foods. You know, it takes a tremendous amount of leafy green vegetables to get many calories. That is why it is so difficult to actually overeat on salads. So, meat from whatever source was a priority for Bob and his kind. He needed many calories to survive his very difficult life. Consider also that it takes considerable energy to provide the necessary fuel for brain function, and compared to other animals, Bob had a huge brain. I mean huge. That was good for Bob and good for us, and that's why we're here.

In terms of the plant food group, Bob ate whatever was available including berries, some fruits, and leafy green vegetables. Remember, these kinds of plant foods do not contain very many calories. Starchy carbohydrate foods were not readily available to Bob or his clan and were not consumed to any large degree. Estimates would suggest that probably less than half of his caloric consumption came from the plants. Again, it would take a large amount of leaves to get many calories, so even if plants were consumed daily, they would not contribute much in the way of available energy. There were times, during the cold season, that probably 70%, if not more, of available calories came from animals. The bottom line is this; meat is a natural food for man.

Bob's ancestors probably ate meat that was left over from other animal kills because they had not, at that time, developed much in the way of hunting skills. In other words, they would probably scavenge for their food (I know, yuck!). It may not have been very appetizing, but it was definitely necessary. Scavenging was their main avenue for food, but it was also a source of danger. Early man was probably as much prey animal as he was predator. Talk about stress; consider the prospect of being lunch for a saber-toothed tiger! However, with the passage of time and the wisdom of evolution, Bob eventually became a hunter. Some have speculated that when man began to hunt, it proved beneficial for the evolution of human intelligence. It is possible that the increased demands of that type of problem solving would shift the evolutionary scales in favor of intelligence. This does not mean, however, that hunting increased human intelligence, per se. (So, don't think you can buy a hunting license, get camo-clothing, and go to the woods to increase your I.Q!) What it means is that the cunning hunter survived (because he had meat to eat) to reproduce, passing his genes onto the next generation. The less cunning would find the task of hunting too difficult, and thus would be more likely to not survive to reproduce. I suspect mankind tended to "hybridize" based on the intelligence. That is, the more cunning the hunter, the more successful he was at the hunt. The more successful he was, the more likely he was to reproduce and pass on his genetic cunningness (intelligence) to his offspring, and so on.

Once Bob became a proficient hunter, protein sources provided more and more of his diet. Despite the fact that a large amount of meat was eaten, his dietary fat intake was probably not excessive. It was a different kind of fat. Remember, he was killing and eating wild game. This would produce characteristically lean meat, although that really didn't matter very much. Fat is a calorie rich food, so it delivers much condensed energy. Bob was constantly moving, walking, running, lifting, carrying, and so forth, and he needed all the available energy he could consume. Remember, his instincts told him to eat all that he could whenever he could. This was absolutely necessary for survival. Whether the game animal was lean or fat, it didn't matter; he needed all the calories he could get. Wild game is still a healthy natural food.

Considering that Bob had a difficult time finding adequate food and that he got a variety of strenuous exercise, he probably didn't have Syndrome X. By the same token, Bob probably didn't live long enough to get Syndrome X. His lifespan was about 30–35 years. (Oh, I can hear all the vegetarians out there making noise.) This is not because all that meat was bad for him. It was not. It was because of the harshness of his life and the prevalence of accidental death. Life for Bob and his clan was extremely difficult. There certainly were stressors related to being nomadic. The climate was often harsh, and it's likely that warfare was common. And even though man had learned to hunt, he was hunted as well.

Now, let's fast forward to the Neolithic Period. About ten thousand years ago (approximately 8,000 B.C.) the Agricultural Revolution began. That was the beginning of farming, and this did not happen around the world at the same time. Some areas began farming considerably earlier than other areas. The world was exceedingly large at that time. Up until the Agricultural Revolution, primary plant groups consisted of fruits and vegetables rather than cereals and root crops. The Agricultural Revolution dramatically changed our diets. Now the human diet became rich in large amounts of carbohydrates in the form of whole grains, legumes, starchy roots and tubers, as well as fruits and berries. Even though the carbohydrate intake of man rapidly increased, these carbohydrates were still simple, unprocessed foods that were digested and absorbed slowly, causing almost no serious rise in blood glucose levels. Not that Neolithic man would care. I imagine he was just happy to have plenty to eat.

If we were to transform Paleolithic Bob into Neolithic Bob, we would find that his diet was pretty good. In the Agricultural Era, not only were plant food forms developed and technology improved, but also animals were domesticated and readily available for consumption. This diet provided plenty of protein and slow release carbohydrates. Bob was provided ample amounts of energy for working and didn't suffer much hunger due to the type of food he ate. During this era, carbohydrates became a much larger and more important food source than ever before. With farming, man did not have to continually wander and forage in search of food, so mankind, or at least some groups, could become more stationary and initiate the early developments of civilization.

Farming meant that man had learned enough to reproduce various crops. Grains were not the only plants reproduced but in this era they became more popular. With the ability to produce various grains came the early forms of bread. However, this was not the soft, white stuff that you know as bread. These early forms of bread were made from very coarse ground flour and because of that, they were quite good for human consumption. The bread consumed in the Roman Empire, the bread consumed by King David, and all early breads were whole grain, low GI carbohydrates that were very nutritious. Even the bread that George Washington had at the end of his day was nutritious. I can see it now—Ol' George would come home after a long day on the Delaware and Martha would have whipped up a big loaf of whole wheat bread for him to have for dinner. (Obviously, it didn't help his teeth much, but that's another story).

Up until the nineteenth century, meal was ground between two stones. One stone was stationary, while the other stone rotated. It produced very coarse ground flour that included the husk (bran) and embryo (germ), as well as the endosperm (starch). The fiber and the fat present in this kind of flour made it a low GI carbohydrate. This flour was an excellent food, and it was, of course, not the only food available. Bread may have been the staff of life, but the diet was quite varied. Fruits, nuts, legumes, fish, and meat were also consumed. It was a fairly well-balanced diet. While it varied considerably, depending on locale, man's menu had dramatically increased since the early days of Paleolithic Bob.

THE NEUTERING OF WHEAT

Then our plight began. A European invented the roller mill. The grain was passed between serrated steel rollers, one rotating twice as fast as the other. As a result, the grain kernel was torn apart rather than being ground. This was the beginning of refined flour. With the ripping apart of the grain, the outer layer, or the bran, was easily removed and the germ, or embryo, was easily removed, leaving the endosperm, or starch. This produced a nice, fine, uniform powder that was highly prized. It had a longer shelf life. Unfortunately, after removing the bran and the germ, virtually all the nutritious aspects of the wheat grain were gone. The bran was discarded, which contained most of the B vitamins and minerals. Also, the germ was discarded, and this contained most of the essential fatty acids and vitamin E. What remained was the endosperm or starch. And there you have it; flour was finally produced which was nutritionally void. A nutritious whole grain had been rendered basically useless.

Actually, it even got worse. Modern manufacturers wanted uniform, consistent white flour. Enter chlorine. Yes, chlorine! A poison was introduced to the flour because it does two things. First, it bleaches the flour, destroying the yellow pigments that are natural to the flour, and then it begins predigesting, or maturing the flour by reacting to the gluten. This predigestion only serves to increase the speed at which it converts to blood sugar. That is, it raises it much higher on the Glycemic Index. (By now you know that is bad). Interestingly, the yellow pigments in the flour that the chlorine destroys are actually carotenes, which your body converts into a very healthy form of Vitamin A. Today, in addition to chlorine, several other chemicals are routinely used in flour manufacturing. These include aluminum chloride and nitrogen dioxide to name a few. Guess what, folks—these ingredients are not *"food."*

Then, around the time of World War II, it was decided to "enrich" the flour. This was an attempt to put back a few of the nutrients it had taken away. It was then that nutritionists and scientists recognized that flour had become, basically, a useless dust, rather than real food. So, flour got back some niacin, some riboflavin, some thiamine, and a little bit of iron. There you have it—"Enriched Flour." (Yeah, right!) Hardly!

To bottom-line it—take a fine old grain and strip it of eleven vitamins and half a dozen significant minerals; then strip it of its fatty acids; then add back three B-vitamins and minerals and what have you got? "Enriched Flour." Basically, "Enriched Flour" is an extremely high glycemic carbohydrate, void of much real nutrition. It would be more appropriately termed "neutered flour." I don't think Bob would have recognized "Enriched Flour" as *"food"* at all. However, it would have probably made a pretty good foot powder, which I'm sure Bob would have, undoubtedly, enjoyed.

In summary, we began eating large quantities of meat along with low glycemic carbohydrates in the form of fruits, vegetables, and leaves. With the Agricultural Revolution we ate unprocessed carbohydrates that were digested and absorbed slowly in the forms of whole grains, vegetables and fruits. We also had ample amounts of meat protein at that time, too. Finally, with the refinement in the milling process that rendered wheat almost nutritionally useless, we have reached an era where we must look at our diet. Unfortunately, enriched flour has found its way into so many products. Consider also the fact that refined sugar is a very popular ingredient in many prepared foods. High glycemic value, you ask? You bet! Most crackers, some chips, breads, rolls, pastries, cakes, and cookies—all contain large quantities of enriched flour, and of course, sweets have refined sugar. Now, from all of this, let's consider the popular breakfast dish—the donut (yes, that jelly donut I mentioned earlier). Here, we have the potential for some fairly large quantities of fat, combined with a large amount of enriched flour and high quantities of refined sugar. Now you know why I said it wasn't *"food,"* and why I don't think Bob would identify this as *"food"* either. Basically, what I'm saying here is that our modern, hurried, convenient diet is a long way from the natural foods we were meant to eat. Many of our health problems are a reflection of an unnatural diet. This impacts us physically and emotionally.

CHAPTER 5

The Balanced Diet

PLEASE READ THESE NEXT TWO SENTENCES OUT LOUD. *This is not a high carbohydrate–low fat diet. This is not a high protein–low carbohydrate diet.* There are plenty of the latter around and they just don't set well with me. I guess it's because I know that many carbohydrates are, in fact, "food." In fact, many carbohydrates are **really** "good food." Hopefully, this nutritional plan will represent a balance. That is, good protein, good carbohydrates, and good fats that provide real, usable food for the human body. We need all the macronutrients in a healthy diet. There is no question about it; they all are extremely important in nutrition.

THE DIETER'S MAZE

Remember earlier that I said that diets don't work? However, you can sensibly lose weight if you approach it differently. I think it is best to think of it as adding into your daily consumption some good-tasting, healthy food while leaving off some calorie dense, unhealthy food. For any dietary plan to be successful, you, the dieter, have to be able to stick to it. Any diet that leaves you hungry will fail. Any diet that is too restrictive in terms of food items will fail. Over the years there have been many, many diets that have, in fact, had successful initial weight loss. In spite of the fact that they have been successful with initial weight loss, the vast majority have failed. Why? A person can stay on a fairly restrictive diet for a while and be motivated by their perception of success. However, if the diet is too tough, too restrictive and just not enjoyable, ultimately the dieter will cave in and probably revert back to his or her old pattern of eating. This is why so many people

40

have seen their weight "yo-yo" throughout their life in that dangerous weight cycle. Humans are just not very good at depriving themselves of things that they enjoy. Nor should they be. Life is too short to live inside a small box, with limited options and too many restrictions. Life is restrictive enough as it is. I am a big believer in living life to the fullest with as few regrets as possible. We should enjoy what we eat and enjoy the experience of eating.

Let's try to think very simply. Let's go back to the question of "What should the human animal eat?" We have gained a good deal of insight considering what our ancient ancestors regarded as *"food."* I think we can see that animal proteins are food. I think we can also see that leafy vegetables, fruits, legumes and nuts are also food.

Let's define the word "food" as appropriate fuel for the human body. Using such a working definition, I think we can now see that a donut is not food. In terms of quality, a slice of white bread, a cupcake, a potato chip, a soft drink, and most cookies are not food. Think about it, and you can identify many modern items that are not food. If we lived in a world that eliminated all the items that we could think of that are not food, I wonder if we would even have Syndrome X. Probably not and we probably would not be losing the battle with obesity too. You can readily see the problem. We have a body that's "wired" to eat all we can, whenever we can, in order to survive, but we are at the same time, assaulted from all sides with cheap, readily available "junk food." Most of this consists of bad fats, too much sugar and other high glycemic carbohydrates. If we could eliminate all those items that are not food, we would effectively eliminate many health problems. So much for what's not food—let's now talk about what food really is.

THE MACRONUTRIENTS

Let's take another look at those macronutrients I referred to earlier. The macronutrients are proteins, carbohydrates and fat. In regard to calories, proteins yield about four calories per gram, just as carbohydrates do. Fats, however, yield about nine calories per gram, which make them the most calorie dense of the group. In addition to the macronutrients, we should also consider the effects of fiber, both soluble and insoluble, in terms of health benefits and weight control. Nor can we ignore the benefits of ample amounts of water, because it is hard to lose weight without plenty of water and impossible to be healthy without it. And, from a weight control standpoint alone, we should consider the effects of alcohol. Did you know that alcohol yields about seven calories per gram? Yes, more than carbohydrates and protein and less than fat. Therefore, in any weight management program, alcohol intake needs to be considered. Anything that contains calories is significant.

PROTEIN

Protein is necessary for life. Proteins, which are converted into amino acids, are necessary for growth and repair of *every cell* in the body. There are twenty amino acids. Eight of these are usually referred to as "essential," meaning that they cannot be synthesized by the body, even though they are necessary for life. Therefore, "essential" amino acids must be consumed from outside sources on a regular basis. With careful planning you can probably get the essential amino acids from non-animal sources. (My vegetarian friends assure me of this.) But, since I think that our ancestors did properly identify animal protein as food, so do I. Meat, fowl, or fish make up part of my daily diet—actually, a big part.

"Non-essential" amino acids are the amino acids that the body is able to synthesize. That is, the body can create these amino acids from other proteins that are consumed. While protein is necessary for cell growth and repair, that is not their only function. There is mounting evidence that protein is a necessary step toward improving your immune system. One of the amino acids, tryptophan, appears to be the precursor of the neurotransmitter serotonin. Serotonin plays a major role in many aspects of life and, in particular, mood. Therefore, adequate amounts of protein may be necessary for better emotional functioning. Your body can also burn protein for energy. While I think it is true that carbohydrates and fats are more readily recognized by the body as fuel, protein can, nonetheless, fill the gap when these other macronutrients are in short supply.

On the down side, however, many of our favorite protein sources (meat, eggs, cheese) are partnered with saturated fat. We know that saturated fat is unhealthy and can lead to heart disease and probably a number of other ailments. Don't forget that cholesterol is hazardous to your health and should always be considered. Also, excess protein is difficult to store and the by-products, or waste, from this can cause problems with the liver and kidneys. There has been some controversy regarding this notion. Some researchers are indicating that there is scant real evidence that liver or kidney problems occur in individuals who are healthy, even with excess protein. In the final analysis, excess protein can probably be somewhat damaging to someone who is already compromised by liver or kidney problems. A fairly recent study in *The American Journal of Kidney Diseases* (August, 2002) cites evidence that people on a low carbohydrate–high protein diet might be at an increased risk for the formation of kidney stones. The subjects also had a high acid load in the blood, which can inhibit bone formation. This may just be an extreme circumstance, but I remain quite cautious about too much protein.

As I mentioned earlier, I believe your body readily recognizes carbohydrates as fuel. Carbohydrates appear to be necessary for a number of other things that protein cannot supply very well. It is also my opinion that most of the high protein–low carbohydrate diets available today are just not very good for you. You see, the intake of saturated fats can be dangerously high as well as the demands of the body to burn that much protein for energy. Furthermore, plant matter provides us with much needed nutrition. There is no question about it. In addition to the fiber, vitamins and minerals are present in plants along with other substances that are extremely valuable for optimal health. The phytochemicals in vegetables and fruits have proven to be highly significant in the prevention of many life-threatening diseases. It is beginning to appear that these "non-nutritive" substances play an important role in protecting healthy cells and cell growth. This is extremely important. They are also part of a real food. The benefits of consuming fruits and vegetables are well documented by the National Cancer Institute and the American Cancer Society, so beware of any meat and cheese diet plan. Besides the fact that it probably won't work, you're compromising your health by what you're eating and by what you're not eating.

Okay, back to protein. Depending upon your age, gender, health, and other factors, such as the amount of exercise you receive, the amount of protein each individual needs probably varies considerably. Table 1 illustrates the recommended amounts of protein. Again, there appears to be a good deal of controversy regarding this, and these recommendations may be viewed as approximate. However, it is safe to say that the average, relatively sedentary person needs about .8 grams of protein per kilogram (2.2 pounds) of body weight. For instance an 180 lb. man will weigh about 82 kg. You would then multiply 82 times .8 and this gives you 65.5. This would be the number of grams of protein required per day. Now, endurance athletes such as runners and swimmers, probably require 1.2 to 1.4 grams of protein per kilogram of body weight. Their high endurance exercise causes muscle and connective tissue damage in which the amino acids are necessary for the proper repair and growth. Therefore, if our endurance athlete were a 180 lb. man, he would require between 98–115 grams of protein a day. Likewise, strength athletes (weight-lifters, or others engaged in heavy resistance training) probably require between 1.6 and 1.8 grams of protein per kilogram of body weight per day. Their strenuous resistance training results in muscle cell damage and probably requires the increased amino acids for proper repair and adaptation or growth. Thus, our 180 lb. man, as a strength athlete, would require 131–148 grams of protein a day. That is a lot of protein! It would be very difficult to obtain that much protein from beans and grains. This is one of the reasons that I believe in the consumption of animal protein. Since I am encouraging everyone to embark on an exercise program, adequate protein is necessary, and some guidelines should generally be followed.

TABLE I

PROTEIN RECOMMENDATIONS

Activity Level	Grams of protein per kg body weight	Grams of protein per lb body weight	100 lb person approx. recommend	150 lb person approx. recommend	200 lb person approx. recommend
SEDENTARY	0.8	0.37	37	55	73
ENDURANCE TRAINING	1.2–1.4	0.55–0.64	56–64	82–95	109–127
STRENGTH TRAINING	1.7–1.8	0.77–0.82	77–82	116–123	155–164

Most of us can only utilize, or absorb, a limited amount of protein at one time. This would probably be between 25–35 grams. I think protein consumption in quantities larger than this may largely "waste" the protein, or run the risk of some of the negatives associated with excess protein. Therefore, I am basically advocating the use of protein three to four times a day in quantities of 25–35 grams. That should be adequate for muscle growth and development as well as general body repair, yet not enough to pose any negative health concerns. In a hurried and hectic world it might be difficult to obtain this much protein per day. As a result of this, a wide variety of protein supplements are available at most health food stores. One problem, however, is that amino acid supplements may not be digested or absorbed as readily in the body as proteins coming from natural food sources. Consider also the fact that proteins coming from natural food sources will result in a greater feeling of fullness and satiety that will help control hunger longer. One solution that I think works well is the use of whey or soy protein powder mixed with other foods such as fresh or frozen fruit. This makes a type of protein-fruit smoothie. In this concoction, you get an extra boost of protein that is ingested with other natural food items which appear to increase absorption and satiety and are also convenient for our time-challenged world. They actually taste good too. No, really!

CARBOHYDRATES

As I said, carbohydrate is what the body most readily recognizes as fuel. Just like a car, our bodies need to be refueled regularly in order to run properly. Although we get these fuels from the mixture of carbohydrates, proteins, and fats and, perhaps, even alcohol, carbohydrate is the primary fuel. Just like protein, it too is absolutely necessary to life. Glucose, which is the simplest form of carbohydrate, is essential for the red blood cells as well as the brain and is the main source of energy for the muscles. Carbohydrates form the singlemost important source of nutrition throughout the entire world. Depending on the locale or culture, they represent some 40 to 80 percent of total food energy intake. It appears that the major sources of carbohydrate in all human consumption are: 1) cereals, 2) root crops, 3) sugar crops, 4) pulses (or legumes), 5) vegetables, and 6) fruits. Some carbohydrates are also obtained from milk products.

In summary, carbohydrates are good. They are essential to life. Some of their physiological effects include providing energy, providing a feeling of fullness, improved gastrointestinal functioning, control of blood glucose and insulin levels, cholesterol and triglyceride metabolism, as well as allowing the body to better utilize protein. Also, I cannot overstate the apparent importance of the antioxidants available in fresh fruits and vegetables. These appear incredibly important to the maintenance of health. Shortchanging yourself of these foods could be dangerous. Remember, fruits and leafy green vegetables have been real food for as long as mankind has been here.

The Glycemic Index

Now let me emphasize that all carbohydrates are not created equal. Carbohydrates differ radically in how fast they produce a rise in circulating blood sugar. Here is where we get into the concept of glycemic index. This has become a very popular topic in contemporary times. As mentioned earlier, the glycemic index is a way of gauging the speed at which a carbohydrate is converted to circulating blood sugar. While the concept is simple, the reality is rather complex. A lot of things can affect the speed at which the carbohydrate is converted to sugar. A high glycemic carbohydrate, such as a baked potato or a slice of white bread, when eaten alone, especially on an empty stomach, would be converted to blood sugar fairly rapidly. There is nothing in its way, so to speak, to slow down the process. With no other food to mix with, the high glycemic carbohydrate has a clear shot straight to the absorption mechanisms in the small intestine. However, when mixed with fiber or fat, or even protein, the rate of the absorption is slowed. So, it becomes an issue of not just what you eat, but how it is eaten and with what it is eaten.

So, let's take a look at carbohydrate digestion. This process begins to occur in our mouth where amylase (the starch digesting enzyme in saliva) mixes with the food as we chew it. This amylase breaks down the long starch molecules into shorter molecules such as maltose and malt dextrose or some other sugar. The digestion process can begin before you swallow that mouthful of food. It appears that this breakdown of the starch molecules basically stops once the food hits the acid of the stomach. However, most digestion occurs when the carbohydrate leaves the stomach and reaches the small intestine. The speed at which the food enters the small intestine from the stomach is called the rate of stomach or gastric emptying. Some food components, such as acid or fiber, may slow down the emptying process and, therefore, slow down the overall speed of carbohydrate digestion.

It is in the small intestine that the digestion process of carbohydrate continues. In the small intestine there are huge amounts of amylase to rapidly increase carbohydrate digestion. In addition to this, pancreatic juices are also secreted into the bowel. It appears that the starchier the food, the more amylase hits it and more rapidly speeds the digestive process. This allows the blood sugar to rise rapidly and this brings us back to the importance of the glycemic index (GI).

There are a couple of versions of the GI scale available. One goes from 0 to 100 with glucose being set at 100. Another one goes from 0 to 150. For our purposes, we will use the 0 to 100 index for simplicity. Basically, the higher the number of the carbohydrate on the GI scale, the more rapidly it converts to blood sugar. Some of this concept can be readily visualized.

Imagine a mouthful of baked potato being consumed. Actually, the baking process begins pre-digestion, but that's how we like our potatoes, baked nice and soft. This aids the digestive process. It hits the stomach where the stomach acids attack it after it has already been attacked by the amylase in the saliva. It then passes quickly into the small intestine where the carbohydrate is really "easy" to get to. This causes a concomitant rise, rapidly, of blood sugar levels. This rapid rise in blood sugar is so extreme that your body is unable to use it all. The pancreas recognizes the rise in blood glucose and releases insulin to move this fuel from the bloodstream to inside the cells, where it is needed. But our baked potato has got a lot of carbohydrate and produces a very rapid and significant rise in blood glucose, so the pancreas has to work hard producing enough insulin to handle the amount of sugar present. What then happens is the insulin does its job too well and the blood glucose levels rapidly decline, which signals our brain that we need to eat again. So you see, our potato, or piece of white bread, or any other high glycemic carbohydrate ends up making us hungry again in just a few hours. And high GI foods very likely can make you crave another high glycemic carbohydrate (to help get that blood sugar up again). You can spend all day with your blood sugar fairly rapidly cycling up and down. Guess what, every time it drops, you're hungry again. Here's another problem: many high GI carbohydrates are also fairly calorie dense. That is, they have a lot of calories. That's the cycle and that's why high GI carbohydrates can contribute to obesity. They tend to keep you hungry.

There is another problem with rapidly rising blood glucose. The elevation of blood glucose triggers the pancreas to secrete insulin, and the higher the blood glucose, the more insulin is produced. Insulin has other physiological effects than just dealing with blood glucose. It also affects the metabolism of fat. The insulin activates an enzyme called lipoprotein lipase, which stimulates body fat to store more triglycerides. What a shame! Also, lipolysis is inhibited by the presence of insulin. The insulin stops the body from burning body fat as fuel (not a good thing if you're trying to lose weight). This is another reason to try to stick to low GI carbohydrates. If you slow the speed and magnitude of blood glucose elevations, the insulin response is minimal. All good.

Now, replace that image (the baked potato) with a mouthful of raw apple. The raw apple has more fiber and is more difficult to break down. The cellulose in the cell walls form little barriers to the digestion process. Because of this, it is much more difficult to "get to" the carbohydrate contained within it. Even after it passes from the stomach to the small intestine, it's still a mixture of carbohydrates and fiber that becomes "time released" in terms of giving up its carbohydrate, or starch, and converting it into blood sugar. This produces a slow, low rise in blood sugar that provides excellent fuel for the long run. Also, the pancreas doesn't have to work as hard (doesn't have to produce much insulin). There is no crashing of the blood glucose; therefore, there is no carbohydrate "withdrawal" to cause you to quickly get hungry again.

So, basically, carbohydrates that are high on the glycemic index, or have a high GI, convert to blood sugar rapidly, causing the quick rise and fall of glucose levels. This in turn tends to stimulate the appetite, especially for more high GI carbohydrates. Remember, they also have a lot of calories. Low GI carbohydrates convert to blood sugar slowly, provide great energy reserves and provide a longer lasting feeling of fullness. Keeping it simple, carbohydrates that convert to sugar slowly are a good thing and are really *good food*. Carbohydrates that convert to blood sugar rapidly are not such a good thing and, while still food, they are probably not really good food. This rapid conversion of carbohydrate to blood sugar sets the stage for some potential problems, not just in terms of obesity but also some other real health concerns. *The number one cause of obesity in our country is the over consumption of high glycemic carbohydrates and poor choices with fat.* Understand, also, that unmanaged stress may play a role in the "craving" for these foods. For many people stress causes a craving for sweets, in specific, and for high fat foods, too.

In addition to the cosmetic affect, there is growing research that suggests that the consumption of high glycemic carbohydrates poses a major health risk in terms of diabetes, lipid levels in the blood, high blood pressure and the resulting possibility of coronary artery disease and stroke. (Remember Syndrome X, the metabolic syndrome?) Many of our snack and convenient food items have high GIs. Bread, of course, is high. This is also true for chips, crackers, pretzels, snack cakes, cookies and the plethora of quick fast foods. Remember what I taught you about "enriched" flour? Don't forget it, because it's important.

I think that for thousands of years, man was a reluctant eater of grains. As mentioned earlier, animal protein, leafy green vegetables, fruits, nuts, and legumes were probably recognized as food. I imagine that an occasional handful of ripened grain was also consumed. This, of course, was whole grain. It had the husk (bran), the endosperm (starch), and the germ (the plant embryo). It was very nutritious and healthy. Enriched, or processed flour does not resemble this food. I read food labels and encourage you to read them. If the first or second ingredient in an item is enriched flour, I try to avoid it. It is hard to survive in our culture without getting some of this stuff but, by all means, keep it to a minimum. I'm also somewhat skeptical of whole-wheat flour. I think it really depends on how the wheat is milled or ground. I also think particle size is important. Finely milled whole-wheat leaves the husk and germ so badly "damaged" that they really cannot help but slow down the process of digestion. Coarser, whole-wheat flours are far better. These can provide a lot of fiber to form that "barrier" to slow digestion and, thus, lower the GI.

While the high glycemic carbohydrates are self defeating, low glycemic carbohydrates are excellent food items. Many fruits, vegetables and whole grains fall in this category. While many highly processed carbohydrates such as white flour (again, white flour is somewhat predigested before it ever gets to your mouth) are high glycemic, whole grains and unprocessed fruits and vegetables tend to be low glycemic. There are a wide variety of excellent carbohydrates that have a low GI. Many of the valuable sources of phytochemicals and other antioxidants are low glycemic carbohydrates. A carbohydrate with a GI below fifty-five would be considered a low glycemic carbohydrate. A carbohydrate with a GI of fifty-six to sixty-nine would be considered medium and a GI of seventy or more would be considered high.

The Glycemic Load

In addition to the glycemic index, a new concept for measuring the impact of carbohydrates is called the glycemic load (GL). While the GI tells you how rapidly a particular carbohydrate is converted into blood sugar, it doesn't tell you how much of that carbohydrate exists in a serving of that particular food. That is where the glycemic load is valuable. It assesses the amount of carbohydrate available in a serving of that food. Many times a high glycemic carbohydrate will have a high GL and vice-versa. And, a low glycemic index carbohydrate will have a low GL. The glycemic load is basically the glycemic index of that food divided by one hundred and multiplied by its available carbohydrate content in grams. A GL of twenty or more is high, a GL of eleven to nineteen is medium and a GL of ten or less is low. However, you cannot just assume that because a food has a high GI it will have a high GL. For example, watermelon has a glycemic index of around 72 (on the glycemic index that rates from 0 to 100). However, it has a glycemic load of about five. This makes the watermelon an acceptable food or carbohydrate to consume. Therefore, on your diet plan, you will find some carbohydrates that have a high GI. Those will be carbohydrates that do conversely have a low GL.

Is your head swimming? Okay, take a breath. Here it is: GI = the rate at which the carbohydrate converts to sugar. GL = the amount of carbohydrate in a serving of that food. Okay, better? Abbreviated GI and GL tables appear in Appendix A.

In summary, many carbohydrates are good food. Carbohydrates are readily available to give you energy. However, you need to pay attention to the type of carbohydrate that it is, in terms of its GI and GL. These are the factors that will determine how the carbohydrate is going to affect your body in terms of body fat, general health, and quality of life. Remember, plant foods provide us with those phytochemicals. These substances have been identified as containing properties that aid in disease prevention. In fact, they seem to be linked to the prevention of four of the leading causes of death in the U.S.—cancer, diabetes, cardiovascular disease and hypertension. They also seem to be involved in many processes, including the prevention of cell damage, prevention of cancer cell replication and the decrease of cholesterol levels. They are too good to be ignored.

Okay, you are now probably getting the right idea. You are going to consume plenty of protein paired with low GI and GL carbohydrates several times during the course of a day. As mentioned earlier, you can lower the GI of foods by how they are eaten. For instance, if you consume a higher GI carbohydrate with a lot of fiber, that will slow its digestion and lower its glycemic index. Pairing proteins with carbohydrates will tend to lessen their overall GI. Acids and fats also tend to lower the GI of the carbohydrate. So, it is not just the GI and GL of a particular carbohydrate, but it is what is eaten with it that will impact your body.

Fats

Not all fats are created equal either. Dietary fat, in general, has had an exceedingly bad rap in the past few decades. Apparently, much of this has been undeserved. Of course, fat is higher in calories than either protein or carbohydrates. Proteins and carbohydrates yield about four calories per gram while fats yield about nine calories per gram. Being so calorie dense, there must be some consideration given if you are trying to lose some weight. What I am saying here is that while nuts are good for you, you can't eat a pound of them a day and expect to lose weight. They have just too many calories.

Bad Fats

There is no doubt that cholesterol-rich saturated fats are very dangerous. Fatty cuts of beef and pork should be eliminated or used very sparingly. You should even be a little careful with chicken and turkey, depending on the type. The dark cuts of these fowl have significant levels of fat and cholesterol. Also, most of us know by now that the skin of a chicken is quite fatty and best avoided. You also know that eggs have a relatively high amount of cholesterol and I personally prefer the cholesterol free egg substitutes. However, it appears that some individuals tolerate eggs better than others. If you have cholesterol issues, you should discuss egg consumption with your physician.

To avoid the dangers of saturated fats, we developed polyunsaturated fat. These became very popular and may also be known as the trans-fats. These are the partially hydrogenated oils and have proven to be at least as dangerous as saturated fat. These fats do not exist in nature, folks. It is because they do not exist in nature that they are not *"real food."* The fat molecule has been changed by the addition of hydrogen atoms. This fat molecule, since it does not occur in nature, is difficult for the body to digest. Unfortunately, this is a problem with many of the margarines available today. They contain hydrogenated, trans-fatty acids. These types of fat molecules tend to be more associated with artery disease than even saturated (hard) fats. I think they can be very dangerous. So, after all, it appears butter is better for you than margarine. Hydrogenated fats, or trans-fats, are commonly associated with much of the "junk" food eaten today, including snack foods, potato chips, cookies, and the like. It is very hard to digest this fat and it is strongly associated with vascular disease and other degenerative problems. If it's not real food, it is best avoided. Again, I urge you to read food labels and learn the language so that these fats will not find their way into your diet.

Good Fats

There are many fats that appear to actually be good for us. These are the unsaturated, non-trans-fats found in monounsaturated items such as olive oil, peanut oil, canola oil, and avocado. Remember also that these fats provide "long-legged" fuel supplies. They are great for the long haul. In activities that require a great deal of endurance, these fats are beneficial in providing needed energy. Next to carbohydrates, your body recognizes fat as fuel. All fats are not bad. In fact, many fats are recognized as real food and are essential in human diet. These are called the "essential fatty acids." Other fatty acids can be converted, or synthesized, inside the body. Diet alone provides the only avenue for the essential fatty acids. The monounsaturated fats appear to have many health benefits. There is some evidence that they aid in reducing total cholesterol without reducing HDL (good) cholesterol levels. This was one of the findings from studying the so-called "Mediterranean Diet." Nutritionists began to discover that in many Mediterranean cultures where olives and olive oil were eaten in abundance, total cholesterol levels were not as high as one would expect. In spite of their consumption of fat, there did not seem to be a significant increase in coronary artery disease.

Olive oil and peanut oil have distinctive flavors that are used in cooking, but because of their distinctive flavors, they may not be appropriate for every food item. Canola oil is an excellent choice for multipurpose cooking because it is basically odorless and tasteless. I also like using the canola oil and olive oil cooking sprays. They allow you to stir fry or coat vegetables nicely and can add a nice flavor.

Omega3 Fat

Within the polyunsaturated group of fats, there are some very important fatty acids, the type of fat that is found in marine animals and cold-water fish, in particular. The benefits of fish oil have been demonstrated repeatedly. The Omega3 fat in fish oil appears to decrease sudden deaths, and some studies have shown that eating fish several times a week may prevent heart attacks and strokes. There is also some evidence that Omega3 fats may play a role in mood stabilization, so there may actually be some mental health benefits to eating fish oil. More and more physicians, cardiologists in particular, across the country are encouraging supplementation of Omega3 or fish oil capsules. This is one reason this diet encourages the consumption of ocean fish, particularly the fish from colder waters, such as salmon and tuna, which contain large quantities of these Omega3 oils.

A diet deficient in essential fatty acids can cause serious problems. Skin lesions and rashes have been associated with dietary fat deficiency. These conditions may be caused by the lack of one or more of the essential fatty acids that provide the maintenance of the epidermal water barrier. Also, some gastrointestinal problems can arise from inadequate essential fatty acid consumption. It's no surprise that diets high in saturated fats and cholesterol pose a risk factor for cardiovascular disease. However, did you know that a diet that is deficient in essential fatty acids also appears to be a contributing factor? As mentioned earlier, some essential fatty acids can lower cholesterol levels. One of the most consistent findings is that Omega3 oils can reduce serum cholesterol levels. Omega3's also appear to be helpful in keeping blood platelets from getting stuck together. That's a good thing. That means less risk of clotting and reduced risk for heart attack or stroke. The list goes on and on. Deficiencies in these important nutrients can have an affect on high blood pressure, breast and colon cancer, the endocrine system and the immune system. While fish and marine animals are the highest source of Omega3 fatty acids, egg yolk, meat and organ meats also provide some essential fatty acids. Supplementation with omega3 oils is probably a good idea. While supplementation can be valuable, remember it would take quite a bit of supplementation to equal a grilled salmon dinner.

A remaining good fat comes from many forms of nuts. They appear to be rich in some mono-unsaturated fats that may also prevent heart attacks and strokes. Plus, they give you a tasty snack option. There is one little problem that accompanies nuts. They taste good. They can be a little bit like potato chips in that it is hard to stop eating them once you start. Nuts are a healthy form of fat, but like all fat, there are nine calories per gram of fat. It is fairly easy to overeat nuts and consume too many calories from their fat. That's why I recommend getting a small digital kitchen scale and measuring out one-ounce servings of nuts in plastic bags. If you do this, then you will know when you've had your serving of nuts and when to stop. It's convenient and healthy.

Now you can really see how the diet is taking form—ample protein in divided doses paired with low glycemic carbohydrates and mono-unsaturated and Omega3 fat. This does not mean that every time you eat you should eat a protein, a low GI carbohydrate and a fat. It's just a general rule for most of your major meals. Remember that pairing your carbohydrates with a fat, protein, and fiber reduces the glycemic index. Also, this "partnering up" of your foods is to ensure that you get away from the cultural model that we have of eating one big meal a day, usually in the evening. While some snacks will remain primarily carbohydrates, such as fruit, we want to avoid producing single, high GI carbohydrate meals. Each of the main meals of the day should contain a healthy protein food item. Also, fresh fruits and vegetables should be consumed daily for all the previously mentioned reasons. I cannot stress strongly enough how important the nutrients are in these foods.

CHAPTER 6

The Important "Un"Nutrients

WHILE THE MACRONUTRIENTS ARE THE BUILDING BLOCKS of any nutritional plan, other factors appear to be quite important. These factors include the presence of adequate fiber and water within the diet. Dietary fiber is a significant issue in any weight loss program and is vital to good health. Likewise, an adequate amount of water is essential, not only to weight loss but also in terms of health. Too many people are short-changing themselves on these critical substances. Paying attention to daily intake of fiber and water is a great first step toward better weight management and better health in general.

You also have to consider alcohol. Why? Because it has calories. The calorie content is highly variable, depending upon the type of alcohol consumed. The "mixers" have to be considered also. Since liquor is often mixed with soft drinks or juices, this also increases the calorie content. Beers and wines are also highly variable in terms of calorie content depending upon the type. At any rate, alcohol must be considered given the possible impact of the calories.

DIETARY FIBER

You've heard that fiber is beneficial to your whole life, right? So what exactly is fiber? Dietary fiber is the portion of the foods that we eat that is indigestible by the enzymes in the digestive system. That is, it is not broken down or absorbed from the intestinal tract. You see, it passes right through. Even though it is indigestible, the bacteria of the lower gut, or the colon, may metabolize part of it. Dietary fiber comes from a variety of sources including fruits, vegetables, nuts, legumes, and grains. As you can see, these are plant foods. Remember, humans are omnivores. We are not carnivores, nor are we herbivores. The balance of plant and animal food sources is very important. We know that there are different types of fiber, depending on its source. Some of the fiber found inside of plant cells has been termed "soluble fiber." In contrast to this, some of the fibers found in the cell walls of plants have been called "insoluble fiber." Of course, some plants have more fiber than others. Again, consider the differences in texture between an apple and a potato. Insoluble fiber includes things like cellulose, hemi-cellulose, and lignin. These fibers tend to increase the amount of "bulk" in our intestinal system. Now, this is what your grandparents considered roughage. Naturally, these fibers can be quite helpful in the treatment and prevention of constipation. Unfortunately, this is all most of us know about dietary fiber. It is also valuable in the treatment of irritable bowel syndrome and diverticulosis. Diverticulosis can be a potentially problematic condition and, at its worse, requires surgery. Diverticula are structures in the intestinal wall that form little pouches. These can become inflamed, painful, or even infected. This situation can become quite severe and prevention is much preferred to the treatment. If diverticulosis has already developed, a low fiber diet is prescribed for the patient while the diverticula are inflamed. After the inflammation passes, it is found that a high fiber diet gives better results.

Fiber that has been considered soluble is thought to be useful in reducing blood cholesterol levels. Of course, as previously mentioned, LDL cholesterol levels are associated with coronary artery disease and stroke, so anything that is helpful in the reduction of this risk factor is worthy of attention. The body seems to be able to eliminate cholesterol through the excretion of bile acids. It has been found that water-soluble fiber tends to bind with the bile acids, and that suggests that a high fiber diet may result in increased reduction of cholesterol. Many studies have shown that a variety of fibers are beneficial in the reduction of cholesterol. Increasing dietary fiber is still one of the first courses of action for patients with high cholesterol. Quite a few of my patients have been able to dramatically lower their cholesterol by increasing their fiber intake.

The classification of dietary fibers as soluble or insoluble has become somewhat blurred and the distinction seems to have lost some of its original importance. It appears that some of the fibers that we have traditionally seen as insoluble also have the ability to reduce cholesterol levels, and some of the fibers that we have always considered soluble appear to increase the bulk in the intestine. There is considerable cross-over here. For instance some of our favorite fibers, like psyllium seed husks (this is a fiber commonly consumed in fiber supplements) and oat bran are examples of fiber sources that tend to increase the bulk in the intestinal track and improve laxation, as well as lower cholesterol levels. Just as confusing, some of the soluble fibers are not very effective at reducing cholesterol levels.

Have I made your head swim again? It just may be best to assume that dietary fiber is healthy for us and not get too caught up in assigning it with the labels of "soluble" and "insoluble." In fact, the National Academy of Sciences panel has recommended that the term "soluble fibers" and "insoluble fibers" be gradually eliminated from their terminology. Like many others, I used to think the distinction had significant health implications. Now I don't, but I do believe fiber, whatever kind, is very important to health. The more we know, the more important fiber seems to be.

Okay, now that we have simplified it, let's talk about the benefits of fiber. As already mentioned, it is helpful for constipation and lowering cholesterol levels. Also, increased dietary fiber may, in fact, reduce the risks of some cancers, especially colon cancer. In cultures with fairly high fiber intake, a much lower incidence of colon cancer exists. The basic idea behind this is that, because your digestive system is able to move waste more rapidly through the body, the body has less exposure to any toxic substances that may be present during the process of digestion. Unfortunately, there are a variety of potentially cancer-causing toxins in most people's diet; at least at times. Keeping it moving decreases exposure. You see, decreased exposure means decreased risk.

High fiber diets are also useful for people who wish to lose weight. No question about it. While fiber has no particular calorie input itself, it does provide a feeling of fullness, and remember that fiber often absorbs a great deal of water from its surroundings. That's how it increases its volume weight and provides fullness, so you tend to eat less. Also, fibrous foods often require more chewing and are generally not very calorie dense. Therefore, a person is unable to consume a large quantity of calories in a very short period of time. Imagine trying to get a large number of calories from broccoli or even a pear. You could feel very full fairly quickly from these types of food. This can be quite helpful. Also, most high fiber foods are carbohydrates with a low glycemic index and glycemic load, which means "good food."

Dietary fibers can also help in the prevention and management of diabetes mellitus. Considerable evidence has been accrued that demonstrates that some fibers slow the gastric emptying rates and digestion. Therefore, the absorption of glucose is reduced. Remember earlier we talked about how adding fiber can reduce the glycemic index of the foods you eat? This is an example of that. Fiber content in foods, in a way, renders the carbohydrate (which turns into blood sugar) time released. This is a much better scenario for diabetics. Therefore, keeping a fairly high intake of dietary fiber allows better control of blood sugars. Controlling blood glucose levels is the name of the game here. Fiber has been useful in the treatment of both Type I and Type II Diabetics.

So, how much fiber do we really need? Table II lists the dietary reference intakes for fiber as issued by *The Food and Nutrition Board of the National Academy of Sciences Research Council.* As you can see in the Table, there is some variation according to gender and age. One thing is for sure; most people don't get anywhere near the amount of fiber they need.

Consider here our Paleolithic ancestor, Bob. Now, we know that Bob ate quite a bit of meat, especially when it was available. And, we are pretty sure that Bob didn't eat very much sugar.

TABLE II
DIETARY REFERENCE INTAKES (DRI) FOR FIBER
The Food and Nutrition Board of the National Academy of Sciences
Research Council issued the Dietary Reference Intakes (DRI) for Fiber

AGE	GRAMS PER DAY OF FIBER	AGE	GRAMS PER DAY OF FIBER
Children		**Females**	
1-3 years	19	9-13 years	26
4-8 years	25	14-18 years	26
Males		19-50 years	25
9-13 years	31	51+ years	21
14-18 years	38	**Pregnancy**	
19-50 years	38	<18 years	28
51+ years	30	18+ years	28
		Lactation	
		<18 years	29
		18+ years	29

(Donuts and candy bars were not part of the Paleolithic diet.) But, Bob did eat much fiber. Some estimates run in the range of 80 to 100 grams a day. That's a lot of fiber! I think it would be fair to say that Bob didn't have any major problems with constipation. (It's a wonder he had time to hunt!) All this fiber came from the portion of his diet that was vegetarian. The seeds, foliage, vegetables and fruits consumed contained high amounts of dietary fiber.

So what would constitute a high fiber food? Even among the fruits and vegetables, there is a lot of variability in the amount of dietary fiber. Table 3 illustrates the fiber content in some common foods today.

As mentioned with protein, I think that dietary fiber should be consumed in divided doses. It would be healthier to get 10 grams of fiber three times a day rather than 30 grams of fiber at one time. Eating ample fruits and vegetables throughout the day is an

TABLE **III**

FOOD SOURCES OF DIETARY FIBER

GRAMS OF FIBER ACCORDING TO DIETARY FOOD PORTIONS

Dietary fiber content of selected foods. Am J Clin Nutr *1988; 47:440-7 and Bowes AD, Bowes and Church's Food values of portions commonly used (14th ed. New York: Harper & Row, 1985)*

FOOD	PORTION	DIETARY FIBER	SOLUBLE	INSOLUBLE
Fruits				
Apple	1 Medium	2.9	0.9	2.0
Orange	1 Medium	2.0	1.3	0.7
Banana	1 Medium	2.0	0.6	1.4
Vegetables				
Broccoli	1 Stalk	2.7	1.3	1.4
Carrots	1 Large	2.9	1.3	1.4
Tomato	1 Small	0.8	0.1	0.7
Potato	1 Medium	1.8	1.0	0.8
Corn	2/3 Cup	1.6	0.2	1.4
Grains				
All-Bran	½ Cup	9.0	1.4	7.6
Oat Bran	½ Cup	4.4	2.2	2.2
Cornflakes	1 Cup	0.5	0	0.5
Rolled Oats	¾ Cup Cooked	3.0	1.3	1.7
Whole-wheat Bread	1 Slice	1.4	0.3	1.1
White Bread	1 Slice	0.4	0.3	0.1
Macaroni	1 Cup Cooked	0.8	0.5	0.3
Legumes				
Green Peas	2/3 Cup Cooked	3.9	0.6	3.3
Kidney Beans	½ Cup Cooked	6.5	1.6	4.9
Pinto Beans	½ Cup Cooked	5.9	1.2	4.7
Lentils	2/3 Cup Cooked	4.5	0.6	3.9

excellent way to improve your fiber intake and make sure you get those other important nutrients. Legumes and whole grains are also good sources of fiber. Also, I am not opposed to the use of psyllium husk or other natural fibers as supplements. This can be especially helpful around mealtime when you are attempting to lose weight. Remember that the consumption of dietary fiber with a meal lowers the glycemic index of that meal. This would have a beneficial effect on blood sugars and also aid in weight loss.

WATER

Water is a terrific deal. It is calorie free, fat free, cholesterol free, low in sodium, and it's a natural food. Drinking enough water helps lose body fat, promotes better muscle tone and size, and increases digestive efficiency. It also aids in organ function and is helpful in relieving joint and muscle soreness. Water is also good for your skin and aids in decreasing water retention. Conversely, dehydration is potentially dangerous.

Did you know that most people walk around at all times in some stage of dehydration? Yes, most of us are dehydrated! Did you know that most adults lose about twelve cups of water every day? That's right, and we lose one half to one cup in the soles of our feet. Four cups of water are lost from breathing. Yes, breathing. Perspiration accounts for another two cups of water loss. When you consider that about six cups are lost through urine, you can see that ample water is necessary. However, people just don't, in general, drink enough water. It has been demonstrated repeatedly that drinking ample amounts of water can aid any weight loss program. This is certainly true. Water does help suppress the appetite and enables the body to metabolize fat into energy. Therefore, if your water intake is restricted, it is difficult to burn fat, and it is likely that water retention will occur. But, water is important for a number of other reasons, also.

Water basically serves as part of the body's transportation system by carrying nutrients and distributing them throughout the body. Water also works as a lubricant. It locates in and around body tissues. Many of the body's more sensitive organs including the brain, eyes, and spinal cord are structures that depend on a protective water layer.

Consider this—water is involved in many, if not most, of the biochemical reactions that occur inside of our body. Most of the molecules that make up our body cannot be split without ample water being present. Water is also important in the storage of carbohydrates. The cells in all parts of our body are detoxified by the presence of water. Water is used to carry away the metabolic by-products to the kidneys and eliminates these by-products, or waste products, through urine. We also use the water in our sweat to help dissipate heat through our skin by means of evaporation. Since most people are in some stage of dehydration, many of these processes can be inhibited. This not only decreases our fitness levels but also jeopardizes our health. Water is especially important to people who exercise. Exercise increases our need for large amounts of water. Exercise in hot weather increases our need even more.

How much water? The usual recommendation is for the individual to drink a minimum of eight, 8 oz. glasses of water per day. That's 64 ounces a day. I recommend at least 72 ounces a day. Why not go the extra mile? Better safe than sorry. That may sound like a lot of water, but you can do it. However, as mentioned, if the temperature is hot, or if you're exercising, or both, you will require even greater amounts of water. Exercise, as well as stress, increases the need for ample water to help in the removal of waste products from the cells. Physical and emotional stress increases the amount of toxic substances in the body which need to be removed. So stressors, both positive (exercise) and negative (illness, emotional, etc.) increase the need for plenty of water. Yet, it is possible to drink too much water. Too much water can result in the loss of sodium and important electrolytes in the body. Low sodium levels are referred to as hyponatremia. This does not happen very often. It would take 2 to 3 gallons of water per hour to have too much water! I don't think this is something you have to worry too much about. It would be really hard to drink that much water.

The best indicator for your hydration level, believe it or not, is the color of your urine. (I know girls; once it's out, you don't look back!) If your urine is dark, this could indicate inadequate water in-take. Basically, you want your urine to be nice and clear and of good quantity. Infrequent urination almost always means dehydration. Dehydration is always unhealthy and can completely wreck your attempt at weight loss. I know there are many fluids out there, and many, if not most, of us were raised on something besides water. However, I think you would be well advised to begin substituting water as your primary beverage. Diet drinks have their own set of problems. I am a bit wary of any diet drinks that contain aspartame. Some studies indicate that this can be dangerous for you. There are a few diet beverages that have safer artificial sweeteners, but it is better to be safe than sorry. Just drink water. So try to forgo the sodas, sugary fruit punches, and the like and drink more water. I actually don't use the "sport drinks" any more because I don't think I need the sugar. What about you? Do you need the sugar?

ALCOHOL

Okay, okay—it has no protein, no fat, and very little carbohydrate, so where in the world do the calories in alcohol come from? Well, alcohol, in its pure form, has around 7 calories per gram. Since it has calories, in a way, it is a form of food and has to be considered if weight control is a goal. Of course, the calorie intake varies considerably depending on the kind of alcohol that you drink. Let's take your average to good quality regular beer. It will weigh in at around 130 to 150 calories per pint. "Lite" beer weighs in at about 95 to 105 calories per pint. Dry wine (less sugar) has fewer calories, obviously, than a sweeter wine. A glass of dry wine contains about 106 calories. A glass of sweet, or dessert wine, can add up to as much as 226 calories. So you can figure this—if you drink a glass of wine before dinner, another glass of wine with dinner, and then an after dinner sweet wine, you've added more than 400 calories to your meal. That's as many calories as a small meal itself! You can't do this on a regular basis and lose weight.

How about hard liquor? A double shot of 80 proof contains about 97 calories. A double shot of 90 proof contains about 110 calories. A double shot of 100 proof contains about 124 calories.

But, that's just the beginning. Many times these liquors are mixed with soft drinks, juices, and mixes that are extremely high in sugar. You can quickly double the caloric value by the time the drink is mixed. I guess you could estimate the average mixed drink will weigh in at 200–350 calories. You can see how quickly this could run into serious calorie trouble.

There's even other problems—calories in alcohol tend to be used before any of your stored fat calories will be used. This is terrible! What this means is that when you consume alcohol, your body will stop metabolizing, or using up, whatever energy source is available and begin to use the alcohol for food. Therefore, a beer or two after a work out is an extremely bad idea. At a time when your metabolism is high and you could be utilizing your fat reserves for your energy, what do you do? You come in and have a couple of beers, which stops the metabolism of the fat, and the flab stays right on your stomach. Alcohol is not a very good fuel for losing weight. Also, the sugar in beer, the maltose, has an exceedingly high glycemic index and is readily going to be stored as fat. So, you are not going to convince anybody that beer is on your diet plan!

Let's just take it at this—for the first couple of weeks that you begin the diet plan, leave all alcohol off. As your weight becomes more what you desire it to be, you can experiment with adding in some alcohol, if you wish. Generally, red wine is the best choice. It is fairly well documented that it has some nutrients in it that may be helpful in promoting a healthy heart.

CHAPTER 7

The Grocery List

I SUPPOSE NOW THAT YOU HAVE SEEN the nutrition plan evolve, it will be fairly easy to guess which foods will be on your grocery list. I am going to divide your foods into two parts. I'm going to suggest that you use the "jump start" program to begin your diet, if you are impatient and are just dying to see some fast weight loss. If this is the case, the first fourteen days you will eat foods on the first grocery list. If you don't believe you need to lose weight that quickly, you can pick items and meals from either list. Remember, my main concern here is that you add some good, nutritious food into your diet so there is less "room" for calorie-dense, high GI carbohydrates, and bad fat.

After your "jump start," you will go to a maintenance or duration diet plan, not to maintain your weight (you should continue to lose weight), but the rate of weight loss should slow down. I actually *want* your weight loss to slow down a bit. Remember, you want to avoid the yo-yo type of body cycling that so many dieters experience. We are looking for a sustained weight loss that can be maintained. What many diet critics say is true—initial weight loss is likely from water loss. When you change your diet to the one I am recommending, you will, of course, lose some body fat, but some of that initial weight loss will be water weight. This is that fast weight loss that accompanies the beginning of any diet.

So after the fourteen days of the "jump start," I want you to go to the "duration diet" and be comfortable that you're losing weight at a healthy, reasonable rate. I think this would be in the neighborhood of 1 to 2 pounds a week. It's really far more important that you keep the weight off rather than just losing some quickly. Remember, some people will lose weight more quickly than others. If your weight loss seems too slow at first, please don't get discouraged. Keep in mind that this diet has two purposes. One is to reduce your body fat. The other is to improve your health. By following the diet conscientiously, you will be able to obtain both goals.

Unless otherwise specified, a portion of food is the amount of food that would roughly fill one-quarter of your plate. Salads are the exception and can be as large as you wish. Also, there are many high fiber, low GI carbohydrates that I don't worry about restricting because their glycemic load is also low. These "free" foods include items like summer squashes, broccoli, asparagus, cauliflower, brussels sprouts, green beans and all the leafy green vegetables. There are others, and after a while I think you will get a "feel" for these types of foods because I use them frequently in the meal plans.

Now a word about fruit. I really like most fruits. They are very good for you and are naturally sweet, so they make great snacks and treats. Except for some tropical fruits, which can have too much sugar, most fruits are low GI carbohydrates and good-to-excellent sources of fiber. Actually, with the current trend toward low carb diets, fruits are greatly under-used, and many people are depriving themselves of a tremendous payload of antioxidants, nutrients, and good tasting foods. I usually eat three or more per day, so when in doubt, eat some fruit!

I was eating an apple while sitting on my office patio once a couple of years ago, and an acquaintance walked up to me and said, "You're eating fruit! Man, that's just sugar. Yep, pure sugar. That's not good for you. That'll make you fat!" I tried, to no avail I think, to convince him that the apple was not "pure sugar" and that it would give me a lot of energy, suppress my appetite, and not make me fat. This is just an example of the many misconceptions there are about carbohydrates, in general, and especially fruit.

As I said, I may eat three or more portions of fruit per day. So what is a portion of fruit? I figure a portion is one small to medium apple, pear, orange, peach, or the like; two or three plums or nectarines, depending on the size, and one half to three quarters of a cup of grapes or berries. Like with most other things, balance is important. It is better to have a portion of fruit three times a day rather than you having three portions at one time.

In order to get the maximum benefit from the food you eat, divided doses works better for nutrient absorption and digestion. I really prefer fresh fruit. It's generally available, although some specific fruits may be seasonal. Frozen fruit would be my next choice. I think you should be cautious of canned fruit because of the sugar content. Likewise, dried fruits often contain concentrated sugar because of how they are prepared. To keep it simple, just stick with fresh or frozen.

I'm also crazy about legumes because they are another source of healthy food. Almost any bean or pea you can think of is marvelous. These legumes are also a low GI carbohydrate with good fiber content and the added bonus of protein. They are, and have been, the staple item of diets in many cultures throughout the world. They are extremely nutritious, and the fiber in legumes is helpful in bringing down cholesterol, so they are valuable in cholesterol-lowering diets. A serving size is about one-half cup, and having a serving or two a day would be great. Preparation can be simple or fancy, but legumes are good food. You can make some terrific bean salads or just open a can. Fresh, canned or prepared from dried, legumes are an excellent value for the quality of food provided. I know, I know, they have a reputation for producing a little intestinal gas, so feel free to try the available products (like Beano) that help with that, or just go commando and see who really loves you!

Okay, back to the grocery list. Here are some items to pick up when you are at the store. Remember, we're trying to add these healthy food items into your diet. The more you can handle on a daily basis, the better.

GROCERY LIST FOR "JUMP START"

PROTEIN GROUP:

Lean cuts of beef such as sirloin and top round steak

Lean pork, particularly lean pork chops

Turkey bacon and Canadian bacon

Veal or lamb

Skinless chicken breasts

Cornish game hens

Turkey breasts

Turkey chops

All types of fish and shellfish

Canned tuna in water

Rabbit

Venison

Other wild game, with the possible exception of duck
(There is a lot of fat in duck)

Fat-free or low-fat lunch meats

Part skim mozzarella string cheese

Reduced-fat cheese (such as Provolone, Swiss and Muenster)

Parmesan, Romano, crumbled Blue or Feta cheese

Low fat cottage cheese and ricotta cheese (part skim is best)

Skim milk

Whey protein powder

Hood–Carb Countdown Dairy Beverage

Soy protein powder

Eggs and egg substitutes
(Use the egg substitute if you have Cholesterol concerns)

CARBOHYDRATE GROUP:

All Bran Cereal (Kellogg's) (ConAgra, Inc.)

Hot cereal, apple and cinnamon

Hot cereal, unflavored (ConAgra, Inc.)

Oat bran cereal

Any protein cereal (such as Total Protein)

Brown rice, steamed

Apples

Apricot

Cherries

Grapefruit

Grapes

Kiwi

Oranges

Peaches (fresh or frozen)

Pears

Plum

Prunes

Strawberries (fresh or frozen)

½ cup Watermelon (remember, it has a relatively high GI but has a low GL)

Blackberries

Raspberries

Blueberries

Baked beans

Black beans

Chick peas (and Hummus)

Kidney beans

Sugar snap peas

Soy beans

Pinto beans

Butter beans

Navy beans

Lentils (either red or green)

Snow peas

Any other beans, dried and boiled

Asparagus

Hearts of palm

Mushrooms

Cabbage

Water chestnuts

Radishes

Green peas

Artichokes

Eggplant

Broccoli

Celery

Cauliflower

Cucumber

All leafy vegetables (spinach, turnip greens, kale, etc.)

Peppers—all kinds

Summer squash (such as yellow crooked neck)

Onions

Tomatoes

Zucchini

Winter squash (such as butternut, spaghetti, and acorn)

Okra (not fried, of course)

ACCEPTABLE FATS:

Olives

Sesame oil

Peanut oil

Avocado

Peanut butter (regular only, reduced fat adds sugar)

Pecan halves (1 oz. or about 15)

Olive oil

Canola oil

Lite nondairy coffee creamer

Almonds (1 oz. or about 30)

Peanuts (1 oz. or about 60)

Other nuts (limited to one ounce)

SALAD DRESSINGS:

Olive oil & vinegar is acceptable

Any salad dressing that has no more than 2 carbohydrates per serving; they should be limited to 2 to 3 tablespoons (2 tablespoons, preferably)

TREATS:

Watch out for the carbohydrate count in sugar-free products— 10 grams or more is not a good thing.

Sugar-free fudgesicles

Sugar-free popsicles

Sugar-free gelatin products

Fat-free sugar-free puddings

SEASONINGS:

Any seasoning that does not contain sugar is acceptable at this stage. Please be mindful of salt. I know we all like it, but too much is damaging.

Imitation Bacon Bits (great for salads)

Sugar substitutes (such as Splenda)

BEVERAGES:

Water

Black coffee (or with 2 Tbs. lite non-dairy creamer)

Unsweetened tea
(Sugar substitute is acceptable as a sweetener for both the coffee and tea)

Vegetable juices (such as V-8 or tomato juice – 6 oz.)

(Remember here, I'm pushing water as the beverage of choice.)

As you can see, there is a wide variety of food available to eat, even in the Jump-Start phase. Also, you can see, there are many more carbohydrates than you would imagine. That's because these carbohydrates listed are low, or at least, reasonably low, on the glycemic index and have low glycemic loads. You can enjoy all of these foods and still lose weight. Do be mindful of portion size as discussed earlier.

You will probably notice that the biggest change to your diet is the foods that are not listed. Of course, there are no "fast" foods, fried foods, packaged or prepared foods, or sweets listed. These are certainly off limits. There is also no high glycemic carbohydrates like potatoes, white bread, or any other items that contain enriched flour. Gone are the chips and the crackers. Gone are the calorie dense, cholesterol laden bad fats that not only contribute to obesity, but can also kill you. But, there is plenty of good food to eat. I urge you to follow the grocery list very strictly in order to get all the possible benefits. Not only will you lose weight, but also you will get healthier. A meal-planning guide for the first fourteen days and recipes for the "jump start" phase is located in Appendix B in the back of the book. However, if you just stick to the allowed food items, you can create many meals and snacks on your own.

GROCERY LIST FOR THE DURATION

For the duration of your eating plan, the grocery list includes everything previously mentioned in the "jump start" program, plus the following:

PROTEIN GROUP:

Cheese (any kind – 2 oz.)

Lean bacon (limit to 3 oz. serving)

Lite yogurt

CARBOHYDRATE GROUP:

Healthy Choice 7-Grain Bread (ConAgra, Inc.)

Whole grain pumpernickel bread

100% Whole grain bread

Whole grain pita bread

Whole wheat rye bread

Long grain, brown and wild rice (not the quick cooking type)

Whole-wheat pasta (including linguini, spaghetti, fettuccini, and macaroni – Lower GI when slightly under-cooked)

Sweet potatoes

Taro

Cantaloupe

Pineapple, mango and papaya (limit portion size to ½ cup)

Yams

Carrots

Honey dew melon

Bananas (not *too* ripe—the GI goes up with ripeness)

FATS:

Remains the same

SALAD DRESSING:

Remains the same

TREATS:

KETOslim High Protein Bar (chocolate peanut crisp)

KETOslim High Protein Bar (chocolate raspberry crisp)

Pure Protein Bars (peanut butter)

Pure Protein Bars (chewy chocolate chip)

Pure Protein Cookies (chocolate chip cookie dough, coconut, peanut butter)

Proto Sport Cookie (any kind)

Popcorn (plain or lite butter – limit to 2 cups)

Again, as you can see, the menu is quite broad in this plan. Some of the foods listed probably surprise you. Nonetheless, if you adhere to this regime, you will lose weight and get healthier. Meal plans and recipes for the duration phase of this diet appear in Appendix B in the back of the book. Remember, if you stay with this grocery list, you can be as creative as you would like and develop you own meal plans and recipes.

SUPPLEMENTS

Most nutritional supplements are not going to improve the quality or quantity of your life. If you follow the recommended diet, I believe all of your nutritional needs will be met. The fruits, vegetables, and good quality protein sources will insure that. With that being said, I am going to recommend considering some supplements to your diet. This is because few among us will always eat wisely at all times. Some supplementation may prove prudent.

Vitamin E was once fairly generally recommended. However, more current studies allude to the possibility that taking supplemental vitamin E may be related to an increase in heart attacks or stroke. Therefore, vitamin E is no longer recommended as a supplement. Be assured though, it is needed in your diet. Snacking with nuts is a good way to get your healthy dose of this vitamin. Leafy green vegetables offer another source, so getting enough of this nutrient through diet alone should be pretty easy.

■ **Fruit and Vegetable Extracts**. There are some forms of fruit and vegetable extracts available today. Given the potential importance of the phytochemicals, I think it would be a good idea to use supplementation from these sources. While the jury is still out, it's a matter of "better safe than sorry." Increasing our antioxidant level seems wise.

■ **Aspirin.** If you have coronary risks factors, you might consider a low dose aspirin daily regime. Certainly, discuss this with your physician and see if he thinks this is right for you.

■ **Vitamin B12**. There are a lot of problems that can result from a deficiency in this vitamin. Loss of balance, anemia, memory loss and other conditions are possible. To complicate it more, at times in our life we may lose the ability to absorb this vitamin efficiently from our gastrointestinal tract. It was once thought that the only way to replace Vitamin B12 was by injection. However, it has been found that oral doses, commonly in the 500 to 1000 micrograms a day works well.

■ **Folic Acid**. 400 micrograms of Folic Acid a day is generally viewed as a good idea for your heart and circulation. It may also play a role in cell protection, particularly the cells lining the blood vessels. Also, folic acid reduces the serum concentration of homocysteine. This is a chemical in the blood that can cause narrowing of some critical arteries that circulate blood to the brain and heart. This is not good! Take your folic acid.

■ **Whey and Soy Protein Supplements**. If you are a vegetarian or have difficulty getting your protein requirements met through your meal planning, these supplements offer an alternative for boosting your protein intake.

■ **Omega3 (Fish Oil) Capsules.** It is probably not a bad idea to include some Omega3 supplementation. This is especially true if you are not fond of ocean fish and do not get the Omega3 oils through diet.

CHAPTER 8

Eating Behavior

REMEMBER THE OLD ADAGE, "It's not what you eat, it's how you eat it"? Well, that's not really an "old adage," and, of course, that's not really true. It does matter what you eat. It matters very much what you eat and I've put considerable effort into demonstrating that to you. It also matters how much you eat. Not only that, it is also important how you consume your food and how you schedule it. There are some good rules and tips for helping you control your weight. You can develop some really good habits that will help you apply some structure to your relationship with food that can make you healthier as well as thinner.

FREQUENCY OF EATING

DON'T SKIP ANY MEALS! I mean it! Don't skip any meals! This is a terrible pattern in our culture and is, inevitably, self-defeating. Whenever I have a patient say to me, "I only eat one meal a day" or "I only eat at night," that patient is almost always obese. A good way to get fat and stay fat is to always skip meals. It is self-defeating and unhealthy. Of course, you cannot eat 1,000 calories six times a day and lose weight. I'm not saying that. However, skipping meals is never a good idea. It's not healthy and it will eventually lead to obesity. Your body needs to be fueled or it will start running "rough." You have to put "fuel in the furnace" if you intend to burn fat. We have plenty of evidence now that infrequent eating can undermine your best efforts at weight loss and fitness. Whereas, more numerous and regular smaller meals will aid your weight loss program and prove much healthier. You will feel better and perform better if you eat regularly. Don't skip meals!

BREAKFAST

This is especially true of breakfast. Don't skip it! Breakfast really is your most important meal. You've got to get your body going. It's been asleep all night and its metabolism is sluggish. You've got to feed your body, which also signals to it that food is abundant enough that it can afford to burn some calories, and we want to burn calories. I believe that a good breakfast should include a protein source because this seems to make breakfast "last longer." Studies have been done that essentially prove that a good protein breakfast goes a long way to curb your appetite through much of the rest of the day, so less food is eaten without suffering any real hunger. Egg substitutes are great for breakfast and represent an excellent protein source. They are extremely versatile and can be used for scrambled eggs, omelets, or frittatas. You can even have some Canadian bacon or some lean turkey bacon with it, which adds even more protein. These egg substitutes are not only a good protein source but also can be paired with an acceptable carbohydrate such as the vegetables listed on the grocery list for omelets, frittatas or whatever. Low fat or fat free cottage cheese is a perfectly acceptable protein food item. This can be paired with a low GI fruit for a perfect breakfast.

Another great protein-rich breakfast is a protein smoothie. This is what I frequently have for breakfast, because I'm always in a hurry. A protein smoothie is one or two scoops of whey protein powder and some crushed ice. Blend these ingredients in a blender with a little water for a few moments, and you'll have a tasty, refreshing, and exceedingly healthy breakfast that is great when you are on the go. One scoop of protein powder provides about 25 grams of protein and the carbohydrate content is usually quite low. Not that there's anything wrong with carbohydrates (you know that by now), but on the first stage of the diet plan, you're trying to "jump-start" your weight loss, and keeping the overall calorie count down is important.

The protein powder comes in a variety of flavors and most of them really do taste good. I know what you're thinking, but they really do! I've converted many people who thought protein supplements tasted bad to this quick, tasty, convenient food. This is a great meal for fueling your body and staving off your hunger for quite a long period of time. There are plenty of other good combinations for a great breakfast. Just try to remember to keep the protein content medium to high and the carbohydrate at a low GI.

I have to make one seemingly unusual request—don't drink fruit juice! I know this is an old favorite at breakfast, but if you want the juice, just eat the fruit. Now I'm not saying that fruit juice is unhealthy, because, for the most part, it's not. In fact, I'm a huge fan of fruit, as you know. Most are loaded with antioxidants and are excellent food. However, there is no point in getting a high dose of fructose (even thought it is a "safe" sugar) without the benefits of the dietary fiber that is contained in the whole fruit. Also, it takes longer to chew the fruit than it does to drink the juice; therefore, it gives you something to do in the time it takes for your brain to register food intake. You see, it takes your brain a few minutes to appreciate the fact that you have eaten something. This is why it's a good idea to eat slowly. Also, consider the fact that if you eat the whole fruit, there is a much greater feeling of satisfaction or fullness. This is due to both of the above reasons. The fiber content and the increased time of consumption both contribute to improve feelings of satiety.

Now that I have made my point about eating a good breakfast, let's go back and look again at the whole notion of eating frequently. There are several reasons for not skipping any meals. One reason is that skipping meals may play havoc with your metabolic rate. Your metabolic rate is the speed at which you burn calories, and, of course, it is important to burn as many calories as possible in order to control or lose weight. Eating frequently seems to increase your metabolic rate. It signals your body that food is abundant and your metabolism reacts by burning more calories freely. This is very good. When you skip meals, your body seems to say to itself, "There is no food available. I must be in a state of famine. I should slow down my metabolism to a 'snail's pace' to save as much available energy as possible if I am to survive." So, when you finally do eat, your metabolic rate is relatively low which only increases your chances of gaining weight from the food that is eaten.

Another reason for eating frequently is to avoid hunger. Feelings of hunger are one of the dieters' worst enemies. No question about it. Quite often self-control goes out the window when the dieter becomes very hungry. I think most of us who have been on a diet have had this experience. Hunger tends to yield impulsiveness, and impulsiveness can often lead to poor food choices and over-eating. So, one of the goals of this diet is to keep hunger at bay and to feel completely satisfied with the food that is eaten. This helps insure success. Remember, one of my main tenants is adding healthy foods into your diet, rather than becoming too restrictive. Yes, I want you to drop some empty or "junk" calories, but I want you to have an abundance to eat.

SNACKS

I want you to eat quite a lot. For this reason, in addition to three meals a day, you will, at least initially, receive frequent snacks. The mid-morning and mid-afternoon snacks may not always involve pairing a carbohydrate with a protein or fat. Occasionally, it is acceptable for snacks to be primarily protein. For instance, a low fat, part skim cheese stick can be an appropriate mid-morning or mid-afternoon snack. Sometimes a few slices of turkey breast or chicken breast will make an appropriate snack. It is perfectly acceptable to have a protein smoothie as a snack, especially if your protein intake has been a little low that day.

There are even times when your snack may be primarily a fat. As mentioned earlier, an ounce of nuts make an excellent snack in that it is very satisfying and provides a healthy source of dietary fat. There will be plenty of times when the snack will be a single carbohydrate like a piece of fruit. As mentioned earlier, a piece of fruit provides low GI carbohydrates that are excellent for providing energy, not just quick energy, but energy for a fairly long duration, all that without the risk of gaining any weight. Small, frequent servings of fruit help "fuel the metabolic furnace" and aid in weight loss while you are getting the antioxidant protection from the phytochemicals.

An excellent snack can involve some pairing of food groups. A small piece of cheese and a piece of fruit can make a perfectly good snack. A turkey/cheese rollup, an apple and peanut butter, and numerous other combinations are possible. Snacks are important for satisfying your hunger, preventing you from becoming very hungry and keeping your metabolism high. However, a snack is just that—a snack. Portion size is important. So, try to keep the quantity down and the source and quality of food good. Remember, I have encouraged you to buy small digital kitchen scales for measuring and weighing your food items. I believe you will find them most helpful in keeping the portion size appropriate.

So, three meals a day will be eaten accompanied by two snacks, one mid-morning and one mid-afternoon. There is also an evening treat after dinner before bedtime. As you see, you get essentially six "feedings" per day, three main meals that our culture is accustomed to and three snacks in between. At first, you'll probably have to remind yourself to eat the snack. If you're not accustomed to it, especially if you've been skipping meals, you might not feel hungry at the time for the snack. I think it is a good idea to have a small snack even if you're not hungry. Remember, you are trying to ward off impending hunger problems. Plus, I want your body to become accustomed to frequent feedings for all of the reasons mentioned above.

LUNCH

Because you have had breakfast and a snack, lunch does not have to be a very big meal. Lunch should ideally involve the pairing of the various food groups. A simple example of this would be a salad consisting of greens, such as romaine lettuce, some carbohydrate, such as squash or zucchini, peppers and onions, and a protein source, such as chicken or turkey. I really like to push for a lot of vegetable consumption at this meal. You can eat rather light and still consume a healthy quantity of raw fruits and vegetables with a nice, complex salad. Any good quality salad dressing made with olive oil provides the third group (healthy fats) to complete the meal. You can accomplish the same thing without eating salad by having a small portion (about four ounces) of chicken breast or lean steak accompanied by green beans, a legume, and/or fresh fruit. Just remember to include plenty of those healthy plant foods. Essentially, many combinations are possible for a very satisfying and enjoyable lunch.

When it comes to the mid-afternoon snack, you may find that this is a way to end that mid-afternoon period of fatigue that many people experience. As mentioned before, a protein snack is perfectly acceptable. But, you can also use a combination of the macronutrients to accomplish this. Vegetables, such as cucumbers dipped in hummus, make a delightful mid-afternoon snack that provide some protein, carbohydrate, fat and continue to provide real food from plant sources.

DINNER

The evening meal tends to be one of the most enjoyed meals in our culture. It comes at the end of the work day and is a time for socialization and family. Incidentally, I think the family unit should eat dinner together as much as possible. I imagine eating together far precedes recorded history. I bet our old buddy Paleolithic Bob ate with his family unit, or tribe, also. Basically, dining with loved ones can be a soothing and comforting experience. Therefore, in the sample menus and recipes located in Appendix B in the back of the book, you will find some delicious, gourmet quality dinner suggestions. Again, these will be groupings of the appropriate protein (you will get a little bit more protein here), low glycemic carbohydrate, and healthy fat. With our broad menu of acceptable foods, the evening meal can easily provide satisfaction and a feeling of fullness for everyone, as well as being an enjoyable experience.

And, to top it all off, you can even have some great tasting dessert items, too. There are some wonderful, great tasting ricotta cheese recipes that provide excellent desserts with a rich cheese-cake-like texture and flavor. This late evening dessert item is designed to provide comfort as well as nutrition. Also, some puddings are acceptable, as well as sugar-free Popsicles and fudge-sicles. This would also be a good time to enjoy a small fruit salad. Many of us just need a little "something" before we go to sleep. (I emphasize a *"little"* something!)

DON'T FORGET THE UN-NUTRIENTS!

Throughout the day, don't forget the "forgotten nutrients"— water and fiber. I know I will be repeating myself here, but I really want you to get this.

Water is extremely important to overall health, as well as weight control. Water is one of the main means of detoxifying our body by relieving the cells of their waste products. Drinking a lot of water can also aid in the feeling of fullness and decrease hunger. So, try to forget the sodas and juices, and try to increase your water intake. If you stay with it, drinking plenty of water can very soon become a healthy habit.

Dietary fiber is also very important. If it is difficult to get enough fiber from the fruits and vegetables, a fiber supplement can be taken. Fiber is helpful in that it inhibits the absorption of carbohydrates into the bloodstream. Remember, fiber in fact can lower the glycemic index of any meal that you eat by slowing down the rate that carbohydrate is absorbed. A spoonful of any fiber supplement that contains psyllium, which is insoluble fiber, mixes with the food that you eat and delays the digestive process. This fiber supplement also comes in an easy-to-swallow capsule that proves to be quite helpful and convenient. In short, you can utilize this psyllium fiber to decrease the glycemic index of the food that you eat, as well as a mild laxative.

OTHER TIPS FOR WEIGHT LOSS

Eat slowly! You are more likely to feel full and enjoy your meals and snacks more if you eat slowly. For instance, if your snack is fifteen almonds, eat them one at a time instead of gulping down the whole handful. If your snack is a low fat cheese stick, pull it apart in small pieces, chewing each piece thoroughly and enjoying it. The same is true of meals. As I said, it takes your brain several minutes to appreciate the fact that you have eaten. So, if you are hungry and wolf down a snack or a meal, you may finish the appropriate amount of food without feeling any sense of satisfaction. Slowing down the whole process increases the chance of feeling full and satisfied by the end of your meal or snack. By the same token, watch portion size. If you eat slowly, it is easier to be mindful of the amount you're eating. And remember, with the exception of salad, any food item that covers more than a quarter of your plate is probably a bit too large of a portion. The "quarter of plate rule" is a good estimate of portion size.

Another helpful eating behavior tip is to pre-plan your menu. This can be done a week at a time or a day at a time. Either way, write down what your breakfast, lunch, snacks and dinner menus will be for the following day and make sure that you have the appropriate food items available. When it comes to the main meals, a rule of thumb I use is to have the protein content about equal to or greater than the carbohydrate content. Also, it is important to keep "safe" food items at your disposal at all times. Keep fruits, nuts and other acceptable food items handy. Be sure you keep them at your work place, home and even in your car. Having this "tool" to manage your hunger will go a long way toward ensuring your success. This type of structure is very helpful in adhering to your dietary plan and in meeting your goal. Too often we have the attitude of "oh well, what shall I have for supper?" and this invites us to consume inappropriate items in inappropriate amounts. By the same token, predictability is important. It is advantageous to have breakfast at about the same time every day, as is the morning snack, lunch, afternoon snack, and the evening meal. Many of the meals can potentially be prepared ahead of time to be readily on hand for the next day. This increases the likelihood of your remaining on your diet.

Yes, it is about losing body fat, but it's also about eating for optimal health and fitness. Try to keep your food choices focused on real food, good nutrition, and reasonable portions.

COMMON SENSE RULES

Considering the above, we can evolve some preliminary rules. Post a copy of these so you can review them daily. It might prove helpful to put them on your refrigerator.

1) Don't skip meals. In fact, eat several times a day.

2) Don't drink fruit juices. Eat the fruit.

3) Keep "safe" foods around you at all times so that they are constantly available.

4) Never allow yourself to get hungry and lose self-control. Eat enough to control *real* hunger.

5) Drink at least 72 ounces of water a day.

6) No fast food, at least for now. The exception would be salads as described earlier.

7) No fried foods, at least for now.

8) No sweets.

9) Limit dairy fat. When eating dairy products choose fat free or low fat only. Sometimes, low fat is actually better than fat free because fat free dairy products often contain more sugars.

10) Supplement your dietary intake with some psyllium fiber, not only to reduce the glycemic index of the food but also to aid the digestive process.

11) Eat slowly. Whether it is a meal or a snack, chew slowly and prolong the experience. Give your brain time to appreciate the fact that you have eaten.

12) Structure your eating. Anticipate, plan and make a menu for at least the next day so that your eating pattern will be predictable.

13) Be mindful of portion size.

14) Don't eat out too often, and if you do, try to follow the basic ideas of the diet. And no **BUFFETS!**

PART THREE

INTELLIGENT EXERCISE

CHAPTER 9

Perspectives on Exercise

Yes, it is possible to lose weight by diet alone. Most, if not all, of the contemporary diet plans certainly can produce weight loss without exercise. This diet can too. It is also true that with just exercise alone, you would have a very difficult time obtaining a significant weight loss. You would have to train like a marathon athlete to lose a significant amount of body weight without a diet. However, it is not possible to optimize your fitness and overall health by diet alone. Diet can go a long way toward improving your blood chemistry, body weight, and perhaps help stave off some diseases, but diet has to be combined with some exercise in order to optimize your quality of life. Through the combination of a smart and natural diet, blended with an intelligent exercise program, you will be able to regain capabilities you once had but have since lost. It paves the way for rejuvenation and revitalization. Many of the processes that we view as a "natural consequence of aging" can be stopped and many times reversed. And that's certainly a good thing! Many of those consequences of aging symptoms are actually the consequences of disuse. We can have some power and control here. Let's see what we can do.

WHAT'S OUR BODY SUPPOSED TO DO?

Just as easily as we ask, "What is the human animal supposed to eat?"—we could well ask, "What is the human animal supposed to do?" Consider again our Paleolithic hunter-gatherer, Bob. Bob traveled expansive distances on nearly a daily basis. Some estimates range around 20 miles a day while foraging. That's a lot of walking. You really might be able to lose weight by exercise alone if you did this! Consider, in addition to this, he sometimes had to sprint and jog, as well as throw, lift, and carry. Bob was an active guy! He and his kind were in near constant motion except when asleep. A full range of physical abilities was necessary just to survive. Bob was, in fact, dependent on his strength, speed and stamina daily. These were important tools for survival. Many times these were the most important tools for survival.

Our ancestral roots demonstrate to us the importance of an active lifestyle. If we fast-forward from our stone-age friend to the Agricultural Revolution, you still find people working hard. It's true during this era that some wealthy upper class people had fairly sedate lifestyles, but the majority of people worked hard. This included, again, considerable walking. Prior to the Industrial Revolution walking was one of the preferred modes of transportation. Actually, if you can't afford a horse and buggy, what are you going to do? Many individuals would spend the biggest part of their daylight hours walking. And, again, the demands of daily living also required considerable lifting and strenuous activity. All of this is certainly very different from our present life style where many of us (myself included) do not have to move much in the course of a day's work. By ancient standards, most of us have a fairly sedate lifestyle. Machines today do the majority of really heavy work. Our strength and stamina no longer appear to be a very valuable survival tool. However, strenuous activity is still what our body thrives on. I said earlier that the human body was designed to function best when it works hard. History would suggest that is true.

If we fast-forward again to our current era, exercise research has generally supported the health benefits of vigorous exercise, regardless of age. From childhood through the lifespan, exercise can dramatically improve the quality of life. It's interesting that many of the current studies support fairly strenuous exercise, even for the elderly, if this can be tolerated. That is, the harder you work the more you benefit regardless of age. "Soft" exercise may be better than no exercise, but it is not nearly as beneficial as more rigorous training.

HEALTH AND FITNESS

I think we all view health and fitness as a positive thing. This is something that we wish to have in our lives. Although health and fitness are both good and sometimes related, they are not the same thing. However, both contribute to the quality (and quantity) of life. So what does health and fitness mean?

Health can generally be defined as the absence of any injury or disease and is also generally associated with physical and mental well-being. Health is just that—being "well." Fitness can be defined as the ability to engage in high-level work activities. Fitness is what you can do, and fitness levels are determined by performance. That is, the more fit you are, the more activities you can engage in with a high level of intensity. Increased fitness can contribute to enhanced health through changes in factors like blood chemistry, body composition, and increased bone density, to name a few. Being healthy and fit allows you to be active, and allows you to remain engaged in those activities which you are passionate about, even as you go through the aging process. What this means is improved quality of life. Reclaiming your health and fitness allows you to take back parts of your life that have been lost. It helps you reclaim some joy and meaning in your life.

We've learned a great deal about fitness training in the last few decades. We are now able to design an exercise program that is scientifically based. You can get the maximum amount of results from your investment of time. In spite of the advances in exercise physiology, one thing remains the same; you still have to work hard. That's right, you have to push it. Your results come from the effort you expend. Therefore, the level of your overall intensity is extremely important.

TRAINING STIMULUS

Let me take a moment and introduce a concept here—*Training Stimulus*. The Training Stimulus is the demand that you place on your body to perform work. This can be the length in time or pace of your walking or jogging. It can also be the number of repetitions of the weight lifted or the amount of the weight lifted. You must have an adequate training stimulus in order to obtain the benefits of your exercise. If it's too easy, then it probably won't benefit you much. The demand on your body must be sufficient to elicit the desired response or training effect. The training effect may be stronger muscles, increased endurance, better flexibility, or a combination of any of these. At any rate, the training stimulus is the amount and intensity of the work that is done. This is regardless of the type of exercise you are doing, and it increases as your fitness level increases. You have to continue to "raise the bar," so to speak. If your desired training effect is stronger muscles, increased stamina, or increased flexibility, your training stimulus must be aggressive. That is, in order for your fitness levels to continue to improve, you must always ask your body to do more and more work.

Earlier in this book, I stated that I was not a big advocate of "walk your dog for twenty minutes a day and that will be sufficient," or "occasionally take the stairs instead of the elevator" type of exercise. I think that these extremely mild forms of activity do not provide an adequate training stimulus. You will perhaps see me state this over and over again, but you have to push hard and invest in exercise in order to reap the best benefits possible. If your work is not intense enough, you will not gain the benefits that are possible. Any exercise that is too easy will not work. Therefore, beware of any gadgets or machines that purport to produce a high level of fitness with very little effort. I get so weary of the seemingly endless array of "work out" equipment that promises dramatic results with very little time and very little work. Again, if it is too easy, it won't be effective. That's just not the way the body works. Intensity produces results, and exercise cannot be intense and easy at the same time.

TYPES OF EXERCISE

I will be discussing three different types of exercise. One is, of course, aerobic conditioning or cardiovascular exercise. The benefits of aerobic training have been well documented for years. Aerobic exercise is absolutely necessary for reclaiming the quality of your life. The second is resistance training, or strength training. Just a few decades ago this was thought to be basically a waste of time in terms of your health. This was considered primarily for appearance only. However, research has indicated it is highly beneficial to you on a variety of levels. I think everyone should practice some form of strength training. The health benefits are phenomenal. The third is flexibility exercise to maintain the ability to have a healthy range of motion in the joints. Loss of flexibility is generally considered to be one of those abilities that deteriorate as a natural consequence of aging. I believe we lose flexibility through disuse, not from aging. Flexibility training is grossly under-rated. It doesn't take a huge investment of time, and actually is a pleasant "cool down" after your other exercise activities. It's a tremendous aid in relaxing and just feeling good.

RECRUIT A PARTNER

Everybody is different. I think it is important for each individual to select an exercise program he or she will continue for the long term. Therefore, each person will have a slightly different exercise program or schedule. It is also important to try to enlist the aid of a partner or a group of people to exercise with you. *Generally, I think that a person who exercises with one or more people will have a four times greater chance of continuing with their exercise program than the individual who attempts it alone.* We can all use an occasional "cheerleader." We can all be an occasional "cheerleader." Exercising with others adds an element of "social support" to the activity. This can move your exercise program from the realm of "work" to the realm of "play." Also, the addition of another person makes us more accountable to the exercise routine itself. It is much harder to miss a workout when you know that someone is waiting for you. So, try to recruit another person or two to exercise with you. This can be family members or friends, and will put more of a "fun" element into it and will maximize your chance of success.

SCHEDULING

There is a variety of ways you can schedule your exercise program. Many people find it advantageous to exercise five or six days a week. These near-daily workouts become a great form of stress management for them. They look forward to the workouts and enjoy the sense of well being that accompanies a fairly strenuous workout. Others, however, find it easier to stay with an exercise program that involves only three or four days a week. Either of these ways of scheduling exercise is fine. Those who exercise daily often perform cardiovascular training on one day, followed by a resistance training the next day and so on. Those that exercise three or four days a week generally perform both cardiovascular and strength or resistance training on the same days. A simple routine would be thirty minutes of cardiovascular exercise followed by thirty or so minutes of resistance training. After each workout some general stretching for flexibility is the appropriate conclusion to the workout.

Theoretically, flexibility exercises and cardiovascular exercises can be performed on a near-daily basis without over-training, as long as the intensity is not too high. Resistance training generally requires a longer recovery time because this kind of exercise temporarily "damages" the muscles. Resistance or strength training can be done on a daily basis if the person trains different muscle groups on successive days, thus allowing the freshly worked muscles to recover. This is called *split training* and is a more advanced training technique. For our purpose here, for general fitness, I think strength training should be done two to three times a week with ample rest in between. This will give great results and is not too demanding.

THE HEALTH BENEFITS

As mentioned earlier, this combination of the "Big 3" (strength training, cardiovascular exercise, and flexibility training) offers extensive benefits. Let's review those health benefits:

1. Build and maintain healthy muscles, bones and joints. (Yes, even bones benefit from resistance training. Weight-bearing exercise appears to decrease the bone loss that may occur with aging.)
2. Reduction of body fat.
3. Reduced risk of diabetes.
4. Reduce risk of some cancers including colon and breast cancer.
5. Reduction of blood pressure.
6. Reduction of cholesterol.
7. Reduce the risk of developing, or dying from, heart disease.
8. Reduced risk of premature death.

THE PSYCHOLOGICAL BENEFITS

The benefits of exercise are not restricted to the physical domain. There are a number of very significant psychological benefits of exercise. In fact, it is probably difficult to find a more conspicuous arena that demonstrates the interconnectedness between our minds and our bodies. A few of these benefits are:

1. Improvement of self-esteem and self-confidence.
2. Mental alertness and improved perception and information processing.
3. Increased perception of acceptance by others.
4. Relief from stress and tension. Exercise is relaxing.
5. Frustration reduction and more constructive responses to the disappointments in life.

There is some evidence that brain chemistry is somewhat changed during exercise. Neurotransmitters (chemicals in the brain) such as serotonin, dopamine, nor-epinephrine, and endorphins are known to have strong affects on mood. Exercise helps in reducing feelings of anxiety, stress, and depression and also seems to strengthen the immune system. Twenty different types of endorphins are in the nervous system. The beta-endorphins secreted during exercise have a very significant effect psychologically. They can produce very powerful positive feelings. That's why so many people feel so invigorated and enthusiastic about exercise. Indeed, the psychological benefits *can* be as profound as the physical benefits. Some research suggests that moderate to intense exercise is as effective, if not more effective, than treatment with the current antidepressant medications available. I try to use "prescriptive exercise" in my practice for the management of anxiety and depression and find it extremely valuable as adjunctive treatment.

WHERE AND HOW

Exercise can be accomplished either at home or at a health club or gym. I personally like the idea of going to a health club or gym for a couple of reasons. One is that when you put yourself through the rigors of getting to a gym, dressed in the appropriate workout clothes with all of the equipment available, it "psychologically urges" you to engage in a constructive workout. Second, because of the vast array of equipment available, there is minimal time spent in changing weights or waiting for your partners to complete exercising, thus you can use your time more efficiently. However, in the final analysis it is up to each person to decide whether he or she wants to go to the expense of joining a health club or invest in some minimum equipment for exercising at home. Of course, much of the exercise can be accomplished without much expense at all, except for a comfortable pair of shoes. Push-ups and sit-ups (resistance exercises), running (cardiovascular), and stretching (flexibility) can go a long way toward recapturing health and fitness and can be done with a minimal amount of financial investment. However, I recommend the investment in an organized gym or health club. I believe this drastically increases your chances of continuing your exercise program. It's just too easy to skip it at home. After several months, or a year or so, you may "get over the hump" and be able to successfully exercise intensely at home. If so, fine, but I think you should begin in a gym. Also, there will likely be individuals there who can give you some useful instruction and information if you need it.

DON'T BE A "WEEKEND WARRIOR"—START SLOW!

Do not begin any exercise program without consulting your physician. Certain health problems can, of course, drastically affect the types of exercise and the level of intensity that you can perform. Your doctor is an integral part of your health and fitness team. Get his or her recommendations before you begin. Go slow! To help ensure that you won't "burn out" on exercise and that you increase your chance of success, by all means start out slowly. Many enthusiastic people often begin an exercise program of somewhat "Olympian" proportions only to become sore, injured and basically disenchanted with the activity. If your lifestyle has been fairly sedentary, start very slowly. Remember that any increase in the level of activity that you have normally been engaged in is, in fact, successful and is movement in the right direction. That is, it will provide an adequate training stimulus. This is not a competition. If exercise is, indeed, going to become part of your lifestyle (which I hope it is), you have plenty of time to make all the gains you desire. I think it is fair to say that most of us are not going to become professional athletes. The exercise we engage in is designed to increase our abilities for the activities we enjoy pursuing. We are trying to slow down, if not reverse, the biological clock. Again, folks, it's about feeling good and enhanced health. (Well, looking good, too, doesn't hurt anything!)

The guidelines for exercise that I am going to set forth here are based on the goal of general fitness. These are the guidelines designed to promote overall fitness levels including lower body fat, increased muscle mass, increased endurance and flexibility. See, that even sounds like rejuvenation! After you have achieved your basic foundation of general fitness, you may modify your exercise program based upon your goals. This foundation is extremely important. It's like the old saying, "You can't run before you can walk." I urge you to spend plenty of time building this strong, safe foundation before you launch yourself into more adventuresome endeavors.

After this foundation is well established, you can slowly begin to push toward new goals. For example, if it is your desire to run competitive 5k or 10k races, you would increase your endurance training and, probably, slightly decrease or modify your strength training. However, if you wish to engage in some amateur body-building or improve your power for specific sports, such as soft-ball or masters' track and field events, you might increase your strength training and only maintain your cardiovascular exercise. Probably most of you will not go on to do competitive power lifting or marathon racing. However, you might. Jon, one of my workout partners, has run in several marathons. I have engaged in competitive power lifting. I once remarked to Jon that running a marathon and competitive power lifting were sort of "cool" things to do, but that I doubted they were very healthy. I noted that a study suggested that extreme over-exercise was actually related to a slightly increased death rate. The training stimulus is just too intense. The extremes that you have to push yourself to, to be competitive, place you right on the edge of injury. The in-creased oxidation and possibility of tissue damage exists. I, in fact, severed the biceps tendon in my left arm once at a power lifting competition and had to have it surgically repaired. That certainly slowed me down, but I learned a valuable lesson. You can push too hard. Your body is very intelligent, and you must train your-self to listen to it. It's finding the balance between an adequate training stimulus on one hand and safety on the other. Much of life is finding the balance. I tend to say that over and over again, because it's true. No matter in what arena of your life, balance is important.

If you're generally healthy, after obtaining your basic level of fitness and strength, the sky is the limit. By working intelligently toward your goals, you will be amazed at what you can accom-plish. I have seen some people dramatically change not only their fitness but also their health. I've had patients that have been able to reduce their diabetic medication, hypertension medication and, of course, antidepressant medication. After completing about nine months or so of strenuous exercise, I had one of my patients tell me, "You really can change your life." And, you really can. It takes effort, but it is well worth it. Basically, after you build your foundation, by obtaining a good level of general fitness, you can tailor your routine to meet your specific needs. I can think of nothing more powerful as a weapon against premature aging than an intelligent exercise program. The potential is absolutely amazing.

CHAPTER 10

Cardiovascular
or Aerobic Training

IF YOU ONLY DO ONE TYPE OF EXERCISE, this is the one to do. No
question about it. The benefits of cardiovascular exercise have
been well documented. Most of us are aware that this is an
extremely important type of exercise to include in our lives if we
are to maintain health and fitness. Most likely, when your doctor
encourages you to exercise, this is the kind of exercise that he or
she has in mind. That's because it's so important for your health.
It is one of the most valuable weapons we have in combating the
aging process and protecting us from coronary disease. Not only
does it have the ability to improve your health, cardiovascular
training can make a profound difference in the way you look and
feel.

One of the benefits of aerobic conditioning is certainly a
stronger heart and improved heart function. Consider that it is
also good for the lungs, improves pulmonary function, and it
increases our blood's ability to carry oxygen and increases the
blood supply to the muscles. Also, heart rate and blood pressure
levels will likely drop with proper cardiovascular training. HDL
cholesterol (the good cholesterol) increases with cardiovascular
training as it does with exercise in general. LDL cholesterol and
triglycerides are much better managed with aerobic training than
by diet alone. It also improves our glucose tolerance; that is, it
reduces insulin resistance. Blood glucose drops because it's easier
to get the sugar (energy) into the cell where it is needed. These are
the kinds of things that contribute not only to the quality of life,
but perhaps to the *quantity* of life as well, as we will see.

One of the most impressive studies followed 17,000 male Harvard graduates between the ages of 35 and 74. In general, the study demonstrated that as activity level increased, mortality level decreased. This is convincing evidence that exercise can decrease death rate, period. The implications from this study are enormous. The men that expended around 2000 calories per week (a little under 300 per day, on average) through such activities as swimming, jogging, and brisk walking lowered their overall death rate by 25-33%. In addition to this, their risk of coronary artery disease decreased by 41% when compared to the inactive group. **Forty-one percent!** This is not only significant; it's down right amazing! With this very compelling evidence it's easy to see why cardiovascular training is an absolute "must" in terms of rejuvenation because of its effects on health and fitness.

WHAT IS CARDIOVASCULAR OR AEROBIC TRAINING?

Aerobic training is exercise that involves large muscle groups and is performed over a prolonged period of time. I will use the terms "aerobic" and "cardiovascular" often interchangeably. Basically, any activity that causes the heart rate to be appropriately elevated for a prolonged period of time is, by definition, aerobic. I say "appropriately" elevated because you don't want it to get too high because that could be dangerous. What would happen if you ran a fifty-yard sprint? For most of us, the sprint would leave us huffing and puffing with a very high heart rate. If you tried to continue sprinting, it could prove too large a demand on your heart and you would fail, one way or another. Cardiovascular exercise has the goal of keeping the heart rate in what is called the "training range." This is the heart rate range where cardiovascular fitness improves, and the demand is not so great that you risk injury or exhaustion. It's the range where you are getting an adequate training stimulus *and* can continue the activity for an appropriate amount of time. Considering all of this, you can see that there are many types of aerobic exercise. In general, it usually involves rhythmical, repetitive motion over more than fifteen minutes. However, almost any activity that involves moving the body through space for a long enough period of time is beneficial in terms of cardiovascular conditioning.

The aerobic exercise that most people have been involved in from one time or another is walking. A word of caution about walking—many years ago I asked a cardiologist about how much aerobic exercise was necessary for keeping a healthy heart. He said, "Just a comfortable walk for twenty minutes or so a day." Well, it turns out that he was wrong. While there are some mild health benefits to casual, slow walking, the real benefits occur from prolonged and faster-paced walking. Again, you tend to reap dividends in proportion to what you invest. Yes, there is some benefit to fairly slow, low intensity walking, but not the high level of gains that are possible with a more intense work out. An article published in *The New England Journal of Medicine* indicated that light walking was, indeed, healthy. However, the study also showed that men who walked less than a mile a day had twice the mortality rates of those who walked two or more miles daily. So, basically, the casual stroll just won't get it when you want the real health benefits possible. Again, we are talking about not only the quality of life, but the quantity of life as well.

In addition to walking, aerobic exercises can include running, or jogging, biking, swimming, skiing, rowing, or group activities such as aerobic dance. You can see that there are many possibilities just as long as you keep moving for a prolonged period of time. There are also numerous machines that are extremely helpful in aerobic conditioning such as treadmills, stair climbers, ellipticals and stationary bikes, to name a few. You might want to experiment with different cardiovascular exercises to find the one that you seem to enjoy the most. Remember, it is important to find the exercise you are likely to stay with and continue long-term. If you enjoy the activity, it will greatly improve your ability to be faithful to it. I can promise you that after you begin to gain some endurance, these activities can really be fun. Also, getting back to the importance of the buddy system, a workout partner or friend can help make the exercise fun and dramatically increase your chance of success.

I find it often helpful to cross-train, or switch activities from time to time. I guess I just bore rather easily. I might walk for a week or two and then switch to an elliptical or stair climber for a few weeks. Then I might change to some light jogging for a period of time. This seems to keep the activity "fresh." Sometimes in the same work out I will do two or more activities, such as the elliptical followed by some treadmill or stair climbing. Remember, the goal here is elevated heart rate over an extended period of time, and this can be accomplished in a variety of ways. So even if you have some pre-existing health problems, you can find an aerobic exercise that's right for you. For instance, some people with low back or knee problems find an elliptical trainer is "joint friendly," where other activities, such as running, would not be possible due to pain or the risk of injury. Stair climbers can be pretty intense, but some of my patients with low back pain find this is better for them than treadmills, which for most people are not as difficult. Regardless of the particular exercise chosen, the results will remain the same—increased endurance, lower body fat, improved blood chemistry and better energy metabolism. Remember that any exercise that keeps your heart rate in the training range for fifteen minutes or more is aerobic and can improve your cardiovascular status. The better conditioned you become, the more you will be able to do and the more enjoyable it will be.

HEART RATE

How fast should your heart beat during aerobic exercise? What is your training range? There are several acceptable ways to calculate this. For simplicity sake, I would suggest using the straight-line method of determining your heart rate range. Basically, you subtract your age from 220 and that number is considered your *maximum* heart rate. No one will recommend that you exceed this number. Then, figure around 60 to 75 percent of that number and that would be a good aerobic range for you as a beginner. For example, if you are 50 years old and subtract 50 from 220, that leaves you with 170. This is your maximum heart rate. Figure 60 percent of 170 and you have a heart rate of 102 beats per minute. Similarly, 75 percent of 170 is a heart rate of 127.5 which you would round off to 128. The goal is to keep your heart rate in your "training range" of 102 to 128 over a period of time. That should provide an adequate training stimulus without risk and is a good, conservative range for the beginner. After your conditioning improves, I suggest you push the intensity levels up quite a bit higher than this. A heart rate in this range may seem a bit easy but remember that you are doing it over a period of time. In the beginning, I like to emphasize the length of time over the intensity level. That is, I'd rather see someone walk for thirty minutes than be able to run a quarter of a mile. It's a better training effect. Running a quarter of a mile is difficult but would actually have very little cardiovascular training effect. It's just not enough time to elicit the desired result. A thirty-minute walk, even if rather slow, will produce some favorable results. As your condition improves, you can increase the upper limits to 80 or 85 percent of your maximum heart rate and raise the lower limits to 65 or 70 percent. I don't think it's necessary to push beyond this level, unless you're a competitive athlete.

How long of a period of time should you exercise? I tend to think that twenty minutes is minimally acceptable. I also think thirty minutes is better. If you have plenty of time on your hands and are interested in more rapidly reducing your body fat, forty minutes is even better. Remember, I favor time over pace, especially with beginners, so if you have to slow down in order to keep at it longer, please do so. With that said, remember you have to start with where you are. If your endurance is not very good, just start somewhere. If you have to start with ten minutes, that's fine, just continue to push the amount of time as your endurance increases. If you can increase the time by two or three minutes a week, it won't be long before you are able to hit twenty or even thirty minutes. So work on training time first and then pace after you've gotten the time up. You'll be happier with the results.

I'm a big fan of heart rate monitors. These are the little devices that you strap around your chest, and you wear the monitoring device on your wrist like a wristwatch. They have become relatively inexpensive and usually run between forty and sixty dollars for a basic unit. There's just no point in guessing at your heart rate when can you know precisely where you are with it. When I do cardiovascular exercise, I like to wear a heart rate monitor to keep an accurate reading of my current heart rate and adjust my workout accordingly. I think heart rate should be the primary guide in this type of training. Clearly, it can tell you when to speed up and when to slow down. You can also keep records of your workout times and the average heart rate obtained so you can chart your progress, which I think is a pretty good idea.

As with exercise in general, a good warm-up period is highly advised. Here's what I most often do. I begin slowly to allow my muscles to warm up gradually. I generally just begin walking if I am on a track or using a treadmill. If I am on an elliptical or stair climber, I just move slow and get the blood flowing. Outside, during colder weather, or if I am feeling some soreness or stiffness, I spend more time on the warm up. After a few minutes I pick up the pace a bit until my heart rate gets set to the training range. I usually continue to pick up pace until my heart rate nears 80 or so percent of my maximum heart rate. Then I slow down a bit and watch my heart rate gradually begin to drop. Before it gets to the lower level of my training range, I increase my pace again. This allows me to keep it in the training range that I choose for whatever allotted time I have to spend that day. Sometimes I work out more intensely by keeping the heart rate at the higher level of the range. Sometimes I keep the heart rate lower and spend more time training and try to focus on the "fat burning" goal and may walk for an hour or more. At any rate, I find the heart rate monitor helpful so that I have some objective evidence of what I am doing. Again, while I think twenty minutes is an adequate minimum, I think it is important to spend as many days as we can in the thirty to forty minute range. When you get in better condition, try an hour or more, at least occasionally.

INCREASING THE EFFORT

Remember to take an intelligent approach toward this task. If you have not been doing any cardiovascular exercise for a long time and your endurance level is low, begin with a simple ten minute or so walk. The main thing is to start someplace. If you've spent years doing nothing, this will provide an adequate training stimulus. Just keep pushing the duration of the time that you're walking and your progress will be evident. If the intensity of your cardiovascular exercise is low to moderate, feel free to engage in it on a daily basis. You will not over-train if your intensity level is not too high. In fact, you will get better results faster by doing your cardiovascular training more frequently. You can train aerobically on a near daily basis and get fantastic results. However, if you get some near serious soreness, it's probably your body telling you it is time to take a day off. Remember to avoid extreme over-training because it can be damaging. Recovery is just as important as the training stimulus. Three days a week is the absolute minimum for aerobic conditioning. You will get almost no training effect if you exercise less than this. Training four to five days a week is near optimum for obtaining significant results at a fairly rapid rate.

As you begin your cardiovascular exercising, your body will begin to adjust and adapt to the training stimulus. That is, you will gradually see increases in your fitness level. Perhaps you will notice that it will take longer for you to feel tired. Perhaps you will notice that it will take longer for you to reach your maximum workout heart rate. Exercise does physically stress your body. However, your body accommodates to the stress by becoming more capable of performing that specific exercise. As you gradually increase the stress again by increasing your pace or the length of time that you exercise, your body will accommodate again. Yes, the body is very intelligent. This is how your fitness level will grow. These adaptations are exercise specific. That is, aerobic endurance increases in response to aerobic exercise. This is the only way your aerobic endurance will increase. Aerobic endurance is absolutely necessary for an increase in the quality of your life and will probably increase in the quantity of your life, as well.

EFFECTS OF CARDIOVASCULAR TRAINING

Chronic effects of aerobic training have been well documented and deserve review. Certainly there is better utilization of fat for energy and concomitant loss of body fat. Blood pressures and resting heart rate decreases. Cardiac tissue of the left ventricle wall increases and the size of the left cardiac ventricle may increase. Cardiac output and stroke volume increases, as does coronary circulation, and there is an increase in the diameter of the blood vessels. What all that means is a more efficient heart! Improvements may be observed in HDL cholesterol (the good cholesterol), reduction in LDL cholesterol and triglycerides, and there may be improved blood glucose levels. Real, measurable changes in your body's physical capacities and blood chemistry will occur. In addition to all of these benefits, aerobic or cardiovascular conditioning tends to illicit an enhanced feeling of well being and improved physical performance in all areas, whether work or recreational activities. This is also an extremely important and efficient stress-management strategy. What all of this means is improved quality and perhaps quantity of life. With all the aforementioned benefits, you can see why I said, if you're only going to do one kind of exercise, this is the one to do. It's too valuable to not do.

By all means, begin slowly. Remember that exercise represents a stressor on your body and your body must have time to accommodate to it. As mentioned earlier, if all you can tolerate is a five- or ten-minute walk, that's fine. In the weeks that follow, just increase that by two to three minutes per week until you have your exercise level up at a minimum standard. It will add up faster than you think. As you continue to improve, you may gradually increase the amount of the stress that is placed on the body and continue to watch your fitness level grow. Remember the intelligence of the body. As you increase the stress on it, your body will accommodate to that stress and will become more capable of doing the work that is demanded of it. As this happens, you will see tasks that once seemed very difficult physically become relatively easy. Your capabilities have dramatically expanded and instead of your endurance gradually eroding with time, you have reversed that process. You will be very surprised how far you can go.

The physical stress placed on the body with exercise is *positive* stress. Negative stress is decreased as a result of exercise, because the exercise itself is an outlet for stress. Remember, uncontrolled, chronic stress is associated with obesity, premature aging, and numerous physical problems. We need all the outlets for stress that we can discover in order to battle the potential physical and psychological problems associated with a stressful life. The interconnectedness of our physical and emotional well-being is conspicuously evident.

CHAPTER 11

Strength
or Resistance Training

EVERYBODY SHOULD LIFT WEIGHTS. Yes, everybody. I really believe that, if you can make yourself do this for a few months, you will be completely satisfied and very motivated to continue, especially if you are working out with one or more people. Strength training can be very satisfying because you can see the results of what you are doing, and if done properly, progress comes at a dramatic pace. You can generally feel and sometimes visually detect changes in your body within the first couple of weeks. Yes, changes in body composition (percentages of body fat and muscle mass) can come very quickly.

THE BENEFITS OF STRENGTH TRAINING

As mentioned before, resistance training (or strength training) has a number of beneficial effects. Certainly, you can improve the amount of lean muscle mass that you carry on your frame. This can also be very helpful as a metabolic aid because muscle is considerably more active than fat on a metabolic level. It takes more calories to fuel muscle than it does fat. This may be one reason why our metabolic rate slows with age. In our sedentary culture, there tends to be a loss of muscle mass with aging. You see, the decline in the percentage of our body's lean muscle mass would, naturally, decrease our metabolic rate and increase our chances of gaining body fat. This does not have to be the case. Also, any weight-bearing activity has a beneficial effect on bone density. This is very important because loss of bone density can be very dangerous as we age. Strength training can also have cardiac benefits, if done relatively quickly, because this would keep the heart rate up. That is, you can potentially have decreases in resting systolic and diastolic blood pressure and positive changes in your cholesterol. Strength training is also helpful in terms of energy utilization; therefore, it can improve glucose intolerance. Along with increases in strength, you also can improve your balance, which aids in most activities. Strength training also appears to stimulate our body's own production of human growth hormone. This hormone is secreted from the pituitary gland and natural production falls off dramatically as we age. Although I don't think human growth hormone is the "fountain of youth," I do think it has some anti-aging qualities such as increased metabolism and improvements in body composition.

One of the things I particularly like about strength training is that you "wear it." Increases in muscle mass often show up as changes in your posture, changes in the way you move, and changes in the way your clothes fit. I think we have all seen people in our day-to-day lives that we know, just by looking at them, that they "work out." That's what I mean by "wearing it." This look has beneficial effects in terms of self-esteem and a generalized feeling of well-being. This, again, demonstrates the inter-relatedness of the physical and the emotional. There are many reasons why we feel better. One reason is that people, in general, respond to you differently when you appear fit and strong. Whether conscious or unconscious, you just receive a more favorable response. Since these qualities are at least somewhat admired, you tend to get some positive feedback, and this can have a tremendous effect on your own self-perception, self-esteem, and mood. Like cardiovascular training, strength training can be a great stress-management strategy. (It's difficult to work out intensely and not feel relaxed.)

As alluded to, since many of us have rather sedentary life-styles, there tends to be a decrease in muscle mass as we age. I don't think this decrease is a natural process of aging. I believe it is simply from disuse. I've seen too many "old" power lifters and shot-putters, and others who have remained quite heavily muscled. Of course, there are a number of individual factors that will determine how much of a particular benefit we get from strength training. Genetics, of course, play a large role in determining how large our muscles will get and how strong we will become. Obviously, men tend to exhibit more muscle growth than women. Most women find this to be a "good thing" because they are not seeking the large growth in musculature to which men may aspire. At any rate, the research strongly suggests that almost everyone can profit from strength training. There have been several studies showing that the elderly gain many of these benefits with some strength training added to their daily routine. Adding and maintaining muscle mass is critical to the rejuvenation lifestyle. Like I said, everybody should lift weights.

THE TRAINING PRINCIPLES

There are a few guiding principles to strength training. It's important to consider these principles when you are developing or changing your exercise routine.

1) The Principle of Gradual Overload. This means that you have to ask your body to perform more work than it does normally in order to stimulate muscle growth. That means training stimulus. Adequate training stimulus must be applied in order for benefits to result. For years I have observed men and women at the gym who basically perform the same workout every time they come in. Not surprisingly, they show very little change in their muscle mass or body fat. I want to go over to them and say, "Add some weight!" and/or "one more rep!" Our bodies, once again, are very intelligent. They only accommodate, or adapt, to the activities that we ask them to do. Therefore, in order to stimulate muscle growth, you must challenge your body beyond its normal workload. This is most commonly accomplished by gradually increasing the amount of weight lifted. However, other changes can stimulate growth as well. Increasing the number of repetitions performed is another way of applying the overload principle. In some specific cases, the velocity that the weight is lifted can be factored in as a way of increasing the overload.

2) The Specificity Principle. This means that gain in muscular strength and endurance will be specific to the exercises utilized. That is, bench pressing will likely increase your bench press ability. It will not, however, improve your leg press ability. Where the goal is general fitness, exercises must be performed that will affect all major muscle groups. That is why it is important how you design your strength-training program. It has to include the whole body.

3) The Rest Principle. This is extremely important to any type of strength training. Sufficient recovery time is necessary between training sessions in order for the muscle to adjust to the stress and adapt to the demands. Basically, resistance training "damages" the muscle fibers. The rest period between workouts allow for the muscles to repair themselves and become thicker and stronger than before. Different types of training regimes utilize different recovery times. For our purposes, we will consider forty-eight hours an acceptable recovery time for resistance training. Some advanced strength athletes do strength training daily or near daily. However, they do not work the same muscle groups on consecutive days. For instance, if the biceps were worked in one training session, it would be several days before the biceps were worked again. For the purpose of general fitness I am going to suggest that workouts be done a minimum of two days a week or preferably three days a week. This will still allow adequate rest or recovery time between workouts.

4) The Detraining Principle. As mentioned earlier, the body adjusts and adapts to the stress or stimulus placed upon it. This allows you to gain muscular size, strength, and endurance by exposing yourself to greater and greater stressors, gradually. By the same token, whenever training stops, your gains will begin to erode. Detraining, or de-conditioning, can usually be seen about two weeks after your strength training ceases.

5) Lastly, the Individualization Principle. This states that everyone tends to respond to the training stress or stimulus in a slightly different fashion. Also, because people may have prior injuries or other conditions, the training program needs to be adjusted or adapted individually. For complicated problems, I would suggest a personal trainer. For our purposes here, the exercises will be very general and well tolerated by most people.

MACHINES VS. FREE-WEIGHTS

Resistance training can be accomplished with almost anything. For instance, you can use your own body weight, as is the case with chin-ups, sit-ups, and push-ups. These exercises are resistance exercises that rely on your body weight as the mass to be moved. When your training is home-based rather than in a gym or health club, you will rely on these exercises as part of your basic routine. Where equipment is involved, I will basically view that as either machines or free-weights.

Machines are found in health clubs and gyms throughout the country. Also, there are a variety of resistance machines available through fitness stores for home use. Machines are great for beginners. As long as you position yourself properly on the machine, they are about as safe as any type of resistance training can be. Machines generally have a fixed plane of motion. That is, the exerciser doesn't have to worry about balance or stabilization of the weight. He or she can focus purely on the effort it takes to move the apparatus through the range of motion. Machines also offer the advantage of being able to isolate muscles in a very strict fashion. Again, they are great for beginners and for isolating muscles for rehabilitation purposes. Machines are a useful way to build a foundation of strength and lifting technique and continue to be useful, even for advanced lifters, at least at times. Also, adding weight is quick and easy (generally just moving the pin to the next heavier weight plate setting). Without spending time changing weights, the workout can progress very quickly and efficiently.

Free-weights are the old-fashioned barbells and dumbbells. There is, undoubtedly, an increase in the risk of injury in using free-weights. However, most people gravitate to free-weights, at least for some exercises. Many of the exercises demonstrated in the workout section will, indeed, be with free-weights. I tend to think that free-weights more closely mimic the activities of daily living where things like balance and stabilization *are* a factor. Because you have to be concerned with balance and stabilization with free weights, they tend to work out a bit more muscle groups per exercise. When I assist people in their training, I usually start them out on machines for several weeks and then add free-weight exercises as their strength improves. Remember, in the beginning the weights are very light because the focus needs to be on proper lifting technique and safety. I don't think it is ever important to emphasize the amount of weight. It is the effort that pays the dividends, not the amount of weight lifted, per se. As stabilization, balance and technique improve, weight is gradually added.

In summary, both weight machines and free-weights have some advantages and some disadvantages. I like to use a combination of them for most workouts, when available. Variety can be very helpful in keeping your exercising interesting. Consider again the advantages of a health club or gym; they generally have a wide array of possibilities for your workout that can eliminate the monotony from your routine.

MULTI-JOINT VS. SINGLE-JOINT EXERCISE

I think this concept is important enough to discuss. As the name would imply, multi-joint exercises require the movement of more than one joint at a time. Therefore, they train or exercise more than one muscle group at a time. Examples of multi-joint exercises include squats, dead lifts, pull-ups, and bench press. Single-joint exercises allow movement of only one joint and predominately train only one muscle group at a time. Such exercises as triceps extensions, calf raises, and isolated bicep curls, are single-joint exercises.

I have a bias toward multi-joint exercises. To me they seem to more closely mimic real life. I think that the lifter learns a certain degree of coordination with multi-joint exercises. Plus, they work more of the body's musculature at one time. Because of this, it takes fewer exercises to train all the muscles of the body. This allows for the exercise session to be made up of fewer exercises and requires less time to complete. Multi-joint exercises subjectively require more effort and tend to be more strenuous. That is, they tend to feel quite intense and induce quite a bit of fatigue. I think this has some advantages, too, in terms of speeding up your metabolic rate and burning more calories.

Single-joint exercises, too, have their advantages. They allow for isolation of particularly weak muscles that need to be emphasized. Because of this, they can also be useful in rehabilitation. Single-joint exercises are useful in the beginning of an exercise program where you really are focusing on building that foundation of strength. Many people have some specific muscles that are relatively weaker than the rest. Single-joint exercises can bring those weaker muscles up to par so that multi-joint exercises can be done more easily.

Because I think most of the readers will be somewhat limited on time, the workout is made up of primarily multi-joint exercises. There are few single-joint exercises demonstrated that will be optional. Some of the exercises that are presented will appear to be single-joint exercises. However, because of the way they are performed they actually pull in other muscle groups and, therefore, are more efficient. My goal here is to present a workout that is time efficient and produces the type of gains that keep people motivated and interested. I want you to very quickly see and feel the difference. Essentially, you can work out 20–30 minutes, with adequate training stimulus, and enjoy all the benefits associated with resistance training.

APPLYING THE PRINCIPLES TO THE WORKOUT

I think the order of the exercises is at least somewhat important. I like to begin with the core of the body. Sometimes when we think of strength training, we forget about the stomach and lower back. The stomach and the lower back represent the very "core" of the body, and it is extremely important to condition them. Remember, a chain is only as strong as its weakest link. In many people, even some who work out regularly, that weakest link is the trunk of the body. Training the core is also important in terms of feeling and looking good.

The abdominal crunch is easy to perform and represents the cornerstone for most abdominal training. I like to alternate sets of abdominal crunches with the "good morning" exercise, or some other lower back and/or gluteus (butt) exercise. This allows you to exercise opposing parts of the trunk. Because there are opposing muscle groups, you can move very quickly from one to the other and back again. In just a matter of minutes you can complete two or three sets of each of these exercises. It helps you warm up and gets you ready for the rest of the workout while you train the core. As the abdominal muscles become stronger, you will want to add more intense training. Something like slant bench sit ups with or without weights can be advantageous. This is because the muscles of the abdomen are no different than the muscles of the arms or legs. They respond to the same kind of training. An increase in muscle size and strength comes from an adequate training stimulus.

Second, I like to exercise the legs. Because leg exercises tend to be quite strenuous compared to exercises for other body parts, it is better to work out the legs when you're fresh. A leg thrust motion is absolutely necessary for strength training. The basic foundation for a leg exercise program is the squat or leg press. These are wonderful multi-joint exercises that directly, or indirectly, hit almost all of the major muscle groups from the waist down. I find them to be absolutely necessary for fitness and health. Leg extensions and hamstring curls are fine if you have the equipment available. Calf-raises complete the leg workout. Sometimes the calves require a lot of work. The muscles may tend to get stronger but sometimes won't increase in size very much. That's not really very important unless you aspire to be a bodybuilder. You will still enjoy the benefits of having stronger calves from doing this workout.

The muscle groups in the upper body are the last to be exercised. There is a lot of variability here in how people work out the upper body. Again, I am aiming toward a time-efficient, yet thorough workout. What that means, of course, are multi-joint exercises. I think what the squat is to the lower body, the bench press is to the upper body. This is an upper body thrust motion. It pulls into play several muscle groups. Although it is primarily seen as a chest exercise, it also works the front part of the shoulders (deltoids) and is an excellent triceps exercise. I think you should probably start with a bench press machine so that balance is not an issue, if one is not available. Then I would begin with a *very* lightweight barbell bench press. The second upper body exercise I would like to recommend is the lateral pull-downs. This is an upper body pull exercise. This is a motion that mimics a pull-up. Of course, if you're strong enough to do pull-ups, you can substitute pull-ups for this exercise, but most people aren't. This exercise will stimulate the muscles in the back, especially the latisimus dorsi and the back of the shoulder group. It also strengthens the muscles in the biceps and forearms and even the grip. Next, move to a basic shoulder exercise, like lateral raises or overhead presses. These, too, stimulate multiple muscle groups. You can finish off with bicep curls and some triceps exercises for the upper arms.

GETTING STARTED

If you have not been doing any strength training, *please* start very slowly. A good starting point for each exercise is to select a weight that you can do fairly easily for ten repetitions. This holds true on all exercises. You must give your body some time to "learn" the technique and become familiar with the stress of the resistance training that you are undertaking. You can turn up the intensity after your foundation has been built and the techniques are well learned.

Begin with abdominal crunches, (Fig. 1) about ten repetitions followed immediately by "good mornings" or back hypers (Fig. 2 & 3). Then rest for one-and-a-half to two-and-a-half minutes and repeat both exercises again. Not only have you begun to exercise the trunk of your body, you are allowing yourself to warm up for the subsequent exercises.

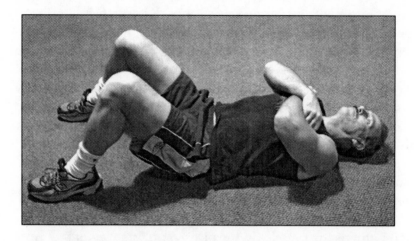

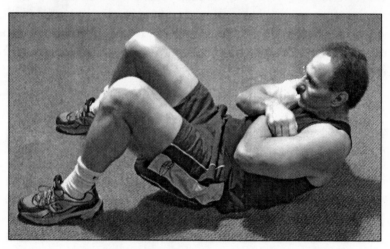

Fig. 1 Abdominal Crunch. You begin this exercise on the floor, knees bent and feet flat on the floor. Using your stomach muscles, you pull your shoulders and upper back off the floor and pause for a second, and then return to the starting position. That is one repetition. Avoid locking your hands behind your head as that can stress your cervical spine (neck).

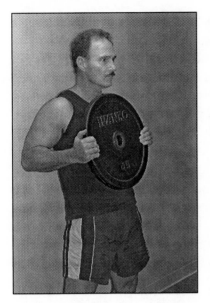
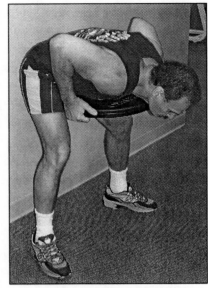

Fig. 2 "Good Mornings." Begin standing, holding a weight plate at your chest. With your knees flexed, bend over, stretching your lower back. Return to the upright position. This is one repetition.

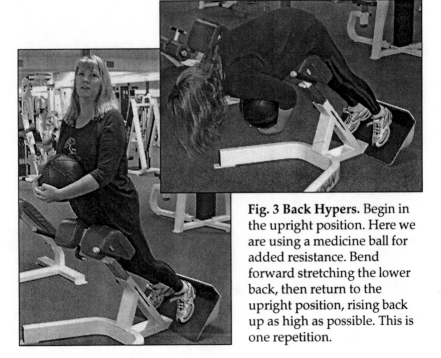

Fig. 3 Back Hypers. Begin in the upright position. Here we are using a medicine ball for added resistance. Bend forward stretching the lower back, then return to the upright position, rising back up as high as possible. This is one repetition.

As you move to your leg workout, I would not start by doing free-weight squats, if you are a beginner. As mentioned, if you do free-weight squats, do them with exceedingly light weight (Fig. 4). Otherwise, try to find a leg press machine and, using the ten-rep rule, do a set of leg presses (Fig. 5). Rest one-and-a-half to two-and-a-half minutes and repeat. If you are going to a health club, finding a leg-press machine will not be too difficult. Another alternative would be using a "hack" squat machine (Fig. 6). If you have a leg extension machine available, after your one-and-a-half to two-and-a-half minute rest, do a set of ten repetitions of leg extensions (Fig. 7). You need not repeat this exercise in the beginning. If a hamstring curl machine is available, do ten repetitions on that (Fig. 8). Repeat the procedure with a calf-raise exercise using the two set, ten-rep rule with rest periods of one-and-a-half to two-and-a-half minutes (Fig. 9).

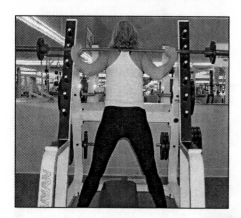

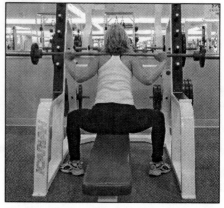

Fig. 4 Squats. For safety sake, I like squatting to a bench or a box. Here, a lightweight barbell is supported behind the neck. Feet are wider than shoulder width for stability. Squat, touching your butt to the bench (without sitting on it, just touch!). Returning to the upright position. This completes one repetition.

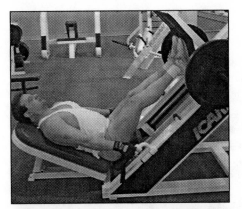

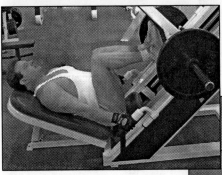

Fig. 5 Leg Press. Begin this movement in the leg extended position. Slowly lower the weight until the knees are, roughly, at a right angle and then return to the leg extended position. This is one repetition. Balance and stabilization are not a problem with this exercise, so it is about the safest of the multi-joint leg exercises.

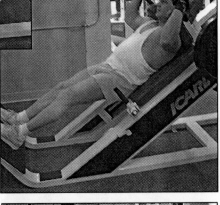

Fig. 6 Hack Squat. Again, begin in the upright position and squat until the knees are at a right angle, and then return to the upright position. This is one repetition. This is a squat motion that is fairly safe for the back.

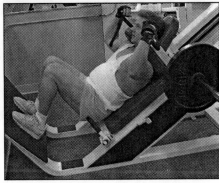

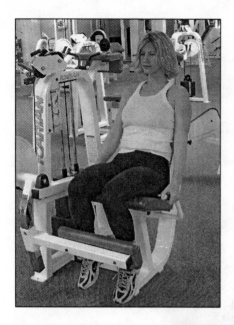

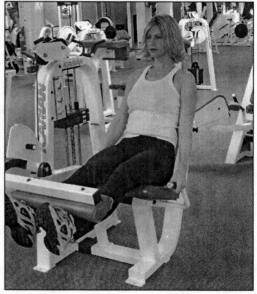

Fig. 7 Leg Extension. This is a safe and simple single joint leg exercise. Just straighten your legs against the resistance and return to the starting position. This is one repetition.

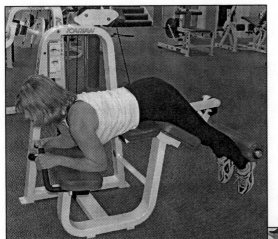

Fig. 8 Leg or Hamstring Curl. Another single joint leg exercise emphasizing the hamstrings. The starting position is with the legs straight. The heels are pulled toward the buttocks and then returned to the starting position. This is one repetition.

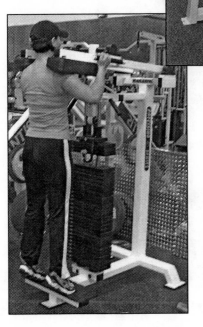

Fig. 9 Calf Raises. There are a variety of calf machines available. They all begin by having your heels lowered and rising up on your toes against resistance. Return to the starting position. This is one repetition.

Moving to the upper body, begin with the bench press. This may be done on a machine initially (Fig. 10), but if a bench press machine is not available and you have to do free-weights, begin with an extra light weight because of the balance and stabilization factors discussed earlier (Fig. 11). Again, two sets of ten repetitions each, with the aforementioned rest periods between sets. Follow the same protocol for the lateral pull-down (Fig. 12), lateral raises (Fig. 13), biceps curl (Fig. 14), and triceps extensions (Fig. 15). This is your basic workout.

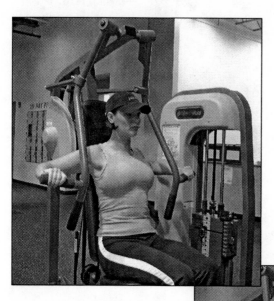

Fig. 10 Bench Press. This seated bench press machine doesn't require balance or stability. It is safe for beginners. You begin with the resistance in the down position and extend the arms to the straight position. Return to the starting position. This is one repetition.

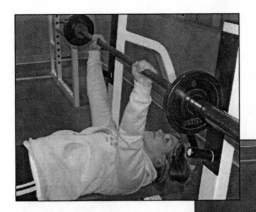

Fig. 11 Barbell Bench Press. Begin with the weight fully extended. Under control, lower the weight and touch the chest. Raise the weight to arm's length again. This is one repetition.

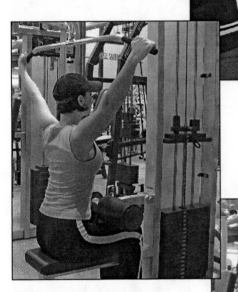

Fig. 12 Lateral Pull Down. Beginning with arms extended, pull weight to top of the chest, and then return to the starting position. This is one repetition. A variety of grips can be used. Here, the wide grip is employed. A narrow grip can be used for variation. The "underhand" grip is also used and tends to emphasize the biceps.

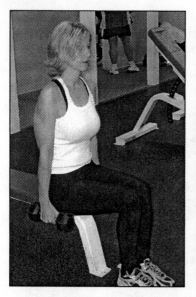 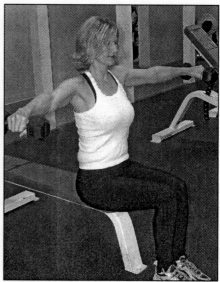

Fig. 13 Seated Lateral Raises. Begin with dumbbells in each hand and hands at your side. With fairly straight arms, raise the dumbbells until your arms are parallel to the floor. Return to the starting position. This is one repetition.

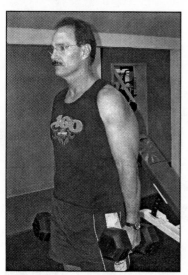 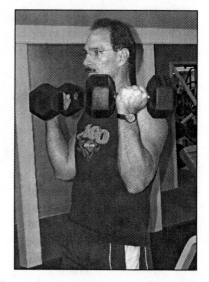

Fig. 14 Biceps Curls. Either dumbbells or a barbell can be used for this exercise. Begin with the weight at arm's length and "curl" the weight toward the shoulders. Return to the starting position. This is one repetition.

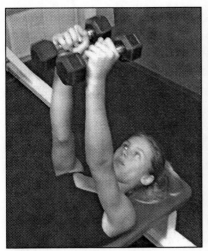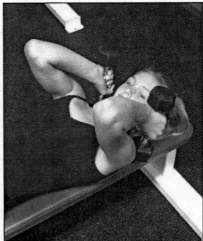

Fig. 15 Triceps Extensions. This exercise can be done with either dumbbells (as shown) or a barbell. Begin with the weight at arms length. Slowly lower the weight until it touches the top of the shoulders, then raise again to arm's length. This is one repetition.

The two-set model outlined above gives you optimum results for minimal time demands. If time is available, I recommend going to three sets after about four weeks of initial training on all exercises. After building the basic foundation of your strength training, this will give you better results. I recommend that this workout be done three times a week. The conventional wisdom has been to work out on Mondays, Wednesdays, and Fridays. This allows for a minimum of 48 hours of recovery time between workouts. This will permit a proper amount of recuperation, which is vital for progress (remember the rest principle). If your time does not allow you three workouts per week for strength training, two workouts will still be advantageous for you in terms of recognizing benefits. I think that two workouts a week is an absolute minimum. If you do go to the two workouts a week, you'll want to divide those equally. For instance, do them on Mondays and Thursdays. You can still get an adequate training effect from this schedule and obviously have ample time for recovery between workouts. With all of that said, the three days a week schedule is still preferable.

After four weeks, or so, your body will have adapted to the new stress (the training stimulus) placed upon it. That is, your body will have already responded to the overload principal and you will be stronger! Your muscles will have begun to "plump out." You've worked out long enough to really see and feel the benefits of resistance training. You've come a long way to building that foundation of strength that enables you to go farther and farther. It is now time to continue the principal of progressive resistance. What I would recommend for all of your basic exercises is to increase the weight lifted by five pounds. You may find that you are still able to do ten repetitions of each exercise. If so, that's fine. However, you may discover that, with the added resistance, your repetitions will drop to eight or so. That's fine, too. Just continue to use that weight until you are able to do the original ten repetitions. After you complete one week of being able to do your original ten repetitions, you will again add weight. You will continue, in this organized fashion, to increase your weight, or resistance, about every two to three weeks, depending on how fast your body is responding. Eventually, you will reach the point when you cannot continue to do ten, or even eight, or perhaps even six repetitions due to the increased weight that you are handling on each exercise. When this happens, it is time to begin a new period or cycle of training. So, the basic rule will be to continue adding small amounts of weight every two to three weeks until your repetitions fall to six or below. At that time you will start all over.

You will have to experiment some and, once again, find a weight that you can fairly easily do for ten repetitions on each exercise. For instance, in the beginning you may have started bench-pressing seventy pounds. When you started, this was the weight you could fairly easily do for ten repetitions. As you begin the second period, or cycle, of training, you will likely find that you can handle a considerably heavier weight for ten repetitions. Perhaps you will start at ninety pounds in this period because this is the weight that you can lift for ten repetitions. Again, you will continue adding weight, about five pounds, every two or three weeks, working up to a point where you can't complete three sets of six repetitions. At that point you will begin your third period of training.

This routine continues in this manner as your strength levels continue to grow. In this way, in a wave-like fashion, you continually challenge your body with an appropriate stimulus (weight) to illicit muscular development and growth. For simplicity, this training system can be summarized as follows:

■ The basic exercises are core training that includes the abdominals and the low back, a lower body thrust motion such as a squat or leg press, upper body thrust motion such as the bench press, an upper body pull motion such as a lat pull down or a pull up, a basic shoulder exercise, and finish off with biceps and triceps exercises. These are the basic exercises.

■ Begin your first cycle with a weight that you can fairly easily lift for ten repetitions for each of the basic exercises.

■ Increase the weight lifted by five pounds every two or three weeks to stimulate muscle development.

■ When the increased weight, over time, causes your repetitions to fall to six or seven, begin a new cycle.

■ In this new cycle decrease the resistance to a weight that you can, once again, complete ten repetitions.

■ Continue with this second cycle by, again, adding five pounds every two or three weeks and continue as above.

■ It may be helpful to keep an exercise journal so you can record and remember the weight that was lifted and when it was lifted.

This type of workout, performed as instructed, will give you the desired affects of strength training. There is no one, best routine for strength training. There are, in fact, many effective training styles and programs for weight training which produce excellent results. If, in fact, you become more serious about weight lifting, there are a number of excellent sources that will outline different systems of training for the serious strength athlete. I particularly would recommend *Periodization Breakthrough* by Stephen J. Fleck, Ph.D. and William J. Kraemer, Ph.D. This is an excellent resource for the serious strength athlete.

The majority of people seeking just a general fitness and increased quality of life will continue this type of program with its simplicity and effectiveness. By the time you have been training this way for ninety days, you will be enjoying your new body and your enhanced abilities to enjoy everyday life. The self-esteem and confidence factors are a bonus and can be quite dramatic. By this time you will easily be able to recognize the stress management component of exercise. Not only do you have a new body, you have a new outlet for stress. I think, at this point, you will see the interconnectedness, or relationship, between your body and your sense of well-being. You will feel more comfortable and at home in your body. This is a fabulous step, psychologically.

While it's not necessarily true for everyone, most people feel the dynamic process involved here—that is, the relationship between what we do and how we feel. Conversely, we can appreciate the connection between what we feel and what we are able to do.

There is a "tumbling domino"-like reaction that can occur with extremely positive results. You see, positive changes in your body yield changes in body image. This in turn yields changes in self-image or self-concept which can have a profound impact on self-esteem, confidence, and overall mood.

This elevation in confidence, mood, and body image can give impetus to more drive and dedication in your involvement with exercise. And the cycle continues. A positive, self-enhancing cycle.

Chapter 12

Flexibility Training

WHY FLEXIBILITY?

UNFORTUNATELY, THIS IS AN OFTENTIMES IGNORED area of fitness training. Basically, flexibility is the ability to move muscles, joints, and bones throughout their full range of motion. The effects of continued flexibility training include improvement in the range of motion as well as improved and more efficient body movement, body awareness, and increased abilities to enjoy the activities of daily living. While stretching may not seem like much "fun" to many of us who work out, it has been shown to improve general levels of physical fitness, reduce muscular soreness, and increase certain performance skills. In some sports, speed of muscle contraction is vital. This is certainly true of sprinting, but also of other sports that involve jumping, throwing, and swinging motions. You see, static or absolute strength doesn't necessarily correlate with speed of muscle contraction or ballistic strength. That's why a big, strong weightlifter can't always throw a ball farther, jump higher, or hit a golf ball further than a physically weaker person. The speed of muscular contraction is critical to many activities like these. Muscles with explosive speed have to be very elastic in order to get that "rubber band"-like snap necessary for many kinds of athletic performances. That's why flexibility is so important in sports training among world-class athletes and can increase the fitness level of the rest of us. It can give us the improved ability to engage in the activities that we love and increase our level of performance in those activities.

Flexibility training has also been shown to improve mental and physical relaxation and to reduce the risk of various joint, back or muscle problems. It is possible that it might even slow the aging process in muscles and joints. Stretching improves the blood flow to the muscles and tissues, and this increased blood flow allows for more oxygen and nourishment to be carried to the muscle group and connective tissue. Flexibility goes hand in hand with the other types of exercise and rounds out your training very nicely.

Stretching is only useful and beneficial to you if it is done properly. Improper technique could result in injury. With proper technique in your stretching, you will enjoy a gradual increase in flexibility. Remember, you don't have to be able to do it like a yoga instructor to profit from it, but you do have to do it correctly. Like just about everything else, learning to stretch correctly is a process. Just do it and keep doing it. Your flexibility will improve with continued practice and patience.

There are various types of stretching. In fact, it appears that many experts have many ideas for the best way to stretch. One form of flexibility training is called active stretching. This involves some degree of "force" to the stretch. Active stretching often involves a partner playing a role in providing the force of the stretch, pushing or pulling their partner's body part to assist in greater range of motion. Ballistic stretching involves the use of momentum in the form of bouncing and very rapid stretching movements. This technique carries the highest risk of injury and I do not recommend it. It could be dangerous, at least to the untrained. Dynamic stretching involves movement also, but this movement is slow, controlled, and rhythmical. I like this technique after some flexibility has already been obtained.

One of the most popular forms of stretching is the static stretching technique. In this technique, the individual moves into a comfortable stretch and holds that position for a desired length of time. This is the safest form of stretching, and still offers a good increase in your range of motion along with the other positive benefits of a flexibility routine. I don't think it is necessary to hold the stretch for too long. Prolonged stretching can, at times, pose a danger and perhaps distort the muscle tissue some. Shorter periods work just as well for the gains we are trying to elicit.

PROPER TECHNIQUES FOR STRETCHING

Stretching cold muscles should not be done. Stretching is best achieved after the muscles have been warmed up. Cold muscles just don't stretch very well and can increase your risk of injury. Like cold rubber bands, cold muscles are a tad stiff and are more easily torn. After muscles are warmed up, they are much more pliable and amenable to stretching. Therefore, I recommend doing the stretching part of your workout as a post-workout, or cool down, after your cardio, strength training, or both. Stretching makes a very nice conclusion to the workout. I know some individuals that do stretch some prior to workouts, and in the "old days" we were taught to warm up with stretching. A better warm up would be some low intensity movement that is controlled and fairly easy which allows the muscle to heat up some with increased blood flow.

Stretching should not be painful. Assume one of your stretch positions and stretch until the muscle feels tight, but still comfortable, and hold for fifteen to twenty seconds and then release and rest for a moment. After a few seconds of resting, resume the stretch but focus on holding it for twenty to thirty seconds. Try to relax as you do this. Avoid the pain threshold and breathe smoothly and deeply. After the twenty to thirty seconds, release that stretch. Now it is time to move on to a different posture and stretch a different muscle group. Flexibility training is not at all demanding in terms of time and is a relaxing, non-demanding process that makes a perfect cool-down.

THE ROUTINE

I'm recommending the following stretch positions: 1) The low back stretch (Figs. 16 & 17), 2) The Achilles tendon stretch (Fig. 18), 3) The abductor's stretch (Fig. 19), 4) The hamstring stretch (Fig. 20), 5) The hip flexor stretch (Fig. 21), 6) The buttocks and hip stretch (Fig. 22), 7) The lateral torso stretch (Fig. 23), and 8) The upper body stretch (Fig. 24). These are basic postures that target all major muscle groups of the body and can be done by most people. Remember, you don't have to be able to do them perfectly in order to profit from them. It is the act of stretching, itself, that improves flexibility, and that's the only thing that will. Remember the specificity principle? If you want to improve your flexibility, you will have to stretch.

Fig. 16 Back Stretch. After kneeling, round out your back as shown and hold.

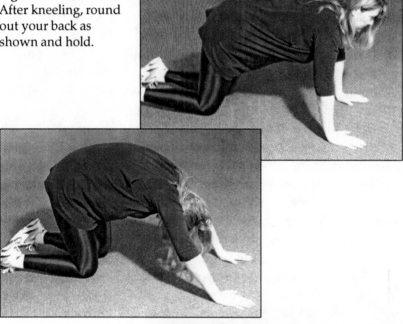

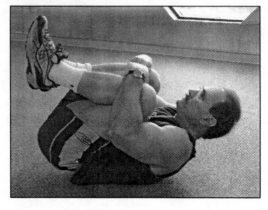

Fig. 17 Back Stretch 2. While lying on your back, pull your knees to your chest and hold.

Fig. 18 Achilles Tendon Stretch. Standing a pace back from a support, lean forward leaving heels on the floor.

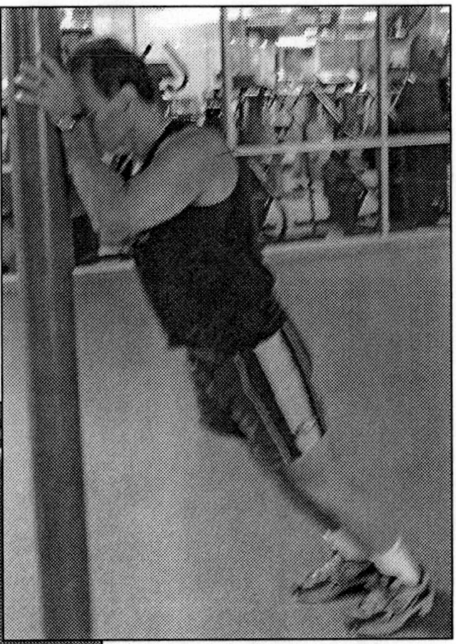

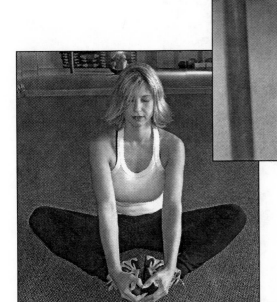

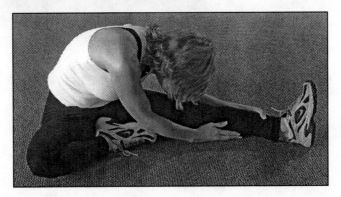

Fig. 19 Adductor Stretch. Sitting upright, with knees bent and soles together, gently push knees toward floor.

Fig. 20 Hamstrings Stretch. Sitting with one leg extended and the other foot against the inner thigh, bend forward, as shown, over the extended leg. Stretch the other side.

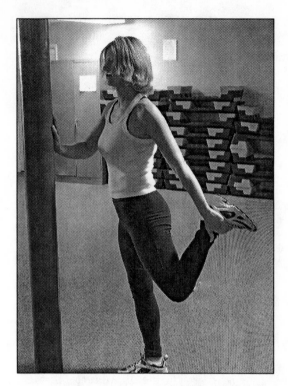

Fig. 21 Hip Flexor Stretch. Stand erect and hold a support. Hold one foot behind you with your free hand. Gently pull the heel toward the buttocks. Then stretch the other side.

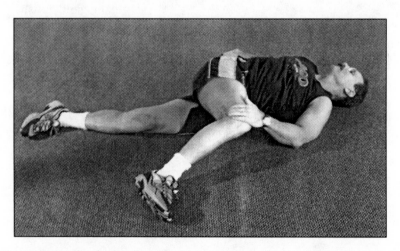

Fig. 22 Buttocks & Hip Stretch. Lie on your back with left leg straight. Bend right leg and pull toward chest. With left hand pull the knee toward the floor, perpendicular to your body. Stretch other side.

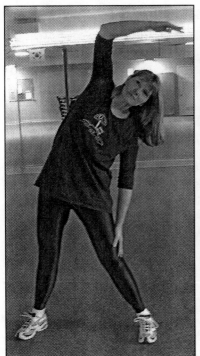 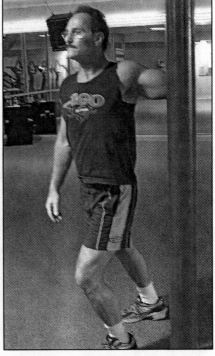

Fig 23 Lateral Torso Stretch.
Standing, extend one hand
overhead and toward the other
side of the body. Stretch the
opposite side.

Fig. 24 Upper Body Stretch. Place
left forearm against a support,
vertically. Gently stretch by
moving the torso forward. Now
stretch the other side.

These flexibility exercises only take a few minutes to do.
Again, they should be done at the conclusion of your workout. If
done on a regular basis, you will very quickly begin to see the
results. Regardless of your age or physical condition, some improvement in flexibility will occur. With that, you will enjoy the
benefits mentioned earlier. Flexible joints have a greater range of
motion and less chance of injury. Increased flexibility means
increased ability in the activities you enjoy. As your flexibility
grows, you will notice the "youthing" quality to it. It allows for an
improved quality of life. Stretching seems to result in increased
body awareness and can be used "meditatively." It's effective in
producing greater physical relaxation and is very helpful as a

stress management tool. I have some friends who are very involved in yoga. They absolutely swear by the benefits of their beloved activity and speak relentlessly about the mind-body enhancement of yoga. I believe them! If you find yourself becoming more interested in serious flexibility training, I would strongly recommend your checking out a yoga center in your area.

All three forms of exercise (cardiovascular, resistance, and flexibility) are good, positive outlets to stress. Yoga is, to me, a very specific technique for stress management. By its very nature and philosophy, yoga joins the mind and the body in "union" and promotes, not just flexibility, but harmony and tranquility also.

PART FOUR

A LITTLE
COMMON SENSE
PSYCHOLOGY

Chapter 13

Stress and Its Management

Okay, let's talk Rejuvenation. I certainly like the sound of that, don't you? I thought so. I have obviously spent a considerable amount of time and effort discussing things that can have a profound effect on your *physical* body. By now you've learned that diet and exercise can reshape your body and allow you to physically reclaim many abilities. You can actually "youth," not just age. Yes, that is one type of rejuvenation. And, if you invest earnestly in your diet and exercise, the physical aspect of your rejuvenation can be quite profound, even dramatic. But guess what? It doesn't stop there. Yes, recapturing physical fitness and health is extremely important. No question about it. Feeling younger physically is a good thing, but what about feeling younger *mentally* or *emotionally*? It's an absolute must. You see, they go hand in hand. Remember the fact mentioned earlier regarding stress and obesity? Stress is a major player in terms of our health and happiness, and the successful management of stress is critical to the entire rejuvenation process. Coping effectively with stress is necessary for your diet and weight control, and it is also vital in terms of beginning and sticking with your exercise program.

I have found that if you don't have the right attitude, philosophy of life, personal psychology, or whatever you want to call it, making major life changes to rejuvenate or embark on any kind of self-improvement is extremely difficult. It is almost like you have to "feel good" to be motivated and be motivated in order to feel good. In many ways this is a cycle. When you feel good and your energy level is high, it is fairly easy to involve yourself in a productive exercise program and follow a good diet. So, your psychological or emotional condition is extremely important in your ability to recapture the quality of life that we are discussing here. Earlier in this book I mentioned that depression could knock you "dead in the water." It certainly can. Depression can render even routine life tasks nearly impossible, much less the rigorous life-style changes we have been discussing in terms of diet and exercise.

Do you remember what inertia is? It goes something like this: "objects at rest tend to remain at rest unless acted upon by an outside force," and "objects in motion tend to remain in motion unless acted upon by an outside force." Well, psychological inertia exists also. When you're eating smart and exercising wisely, you're really in motion, motivation is high, and expectations are positive. It's easy to "stay the course" and continue your self-enhancing life style. Conversely, when you're sedentary, over-weight, and your energy level is low, you are an object at rest and it can be very difficult to muster up enough motivation to embark on the recommendations in this book. That's why I continue to ask you to begin wherever you are with whatever positive changes you can make. Any small, positive change can help "break the ice" on your psychological inertia and initiate the beginning of changes in your behavior and mood that can put you on track to better nutrition, exercise, and a rejuvenation life style. But the key is that you have to start somewhere. Any positive change is a step in the right direction and can result in larger dividends.

Let me ask you something. What's going on in your head? *What are you thinking? How are you thinking?* What do you want your life to be like? Is your life going like you want it to? Are you doing the things that you want to be doing? Is your life full, rich, and satisfying? These are million dollar questions, aren't they? And they are terribly important questions. This is worthy of some discussion.

One thing that is necessary, as you have gathered, is to find an effective means of managing the stress of life. Let's talk about stress for a moment. What do I mean by stress? Stress is anything that requires you to adjust or adapt. Pretty simple, huh? So anything which requires you to respond can be interpreted as a stressor. However, many potential stressors are relatively inconsequential and do not really "feel" stressful. I should mention that, by our definition of stress, many good things in life are stressful, as well. Moving to a new location or even into a new house is stressful. Getting a promotion at work with new responsibilities is stressful. Starting and developing a new relationship may be a glorious experience, but it's stressful by definition. You see, many positives things in life can be stressful. What we are trying to manage is the negative aspects of stress. That is, chronic tension, pressure, anxiety, emotional conflict, and emotional pain. Let me make one point perfectly clear; there is no "cure" for negative stress. We will confront it as long as we live. The only "cure" for stress is the same thing that is the "cure" for life; you got it, **death**. So, managing stress is critical.

When we are first confronted with a stressor, it generally mobilizes us to action. That's good because it means we have been confronted with a problem and are attempting to take action in terms of solving it. Taking action is good, as we will see. However, if the stress becomes chronic because our problem solving fails and the stressor persists, we very often become depressed with some or all of the symptoms that render the situation even worse. As I discussed earlier, depression can produce psychological inertia, so to speak, with sadness, low energy level, poor sleep, decreased motivation and almost no enthusiasm for anything. It can even affect your concentration and memory. With these symptoms, it's easy to see how this would undermine any efforts at improving your health and fitness. Now I think you can more clearly see why stress is associated with obesity and a plethora of other health problems. Stress even appears to play a role in the process of aging. Have you ever noticed a person who has been under extreme stress often appears haggard? It just seems that people enduring chronic stress appear to age more rapidly. Not good!

Yes, psychological stress is not only associated with various physical and emotional disorders, it is also correlated with biological aging, and with accelerated aging come the onset of age-related illnesses. A recent study was presented in the proceedings of the National Academy of Sciences that strongly suggested that psychological stress accelerates aging at the cellular level. While many studies have demonstrated the correlation between chronic, unresolved, or poorly managed stress with poor health, the exact mechanism of how stress affects our health is not understood. However, there has been some recent research that points to the role telomeres play in cellular aging and the potential to develop disease. Telomeres are a DNA protein complex that form a cap over the chromosomes. This appears to promote chromosome stability; however, when cells divide, the telomere is not fully replicated and this leads the telomere to shorten with each cell division. In humans, telomeres shorten with age in all cells that divide. Essentially, telomere length can serve as a kind of measurement of the cell's biological age.

At any rate, this study indicated that chronic, poorly managed stress accelerates the shortening of the telomeres thus accelerating the biological aging process of cells. With the accelerated cellular aging comes the likelihood of developing age-related disorders. Therefore, chronic, unresolved stress appears not only to be able to accelerate biological aging, but also increase the likelihood of developing age-related health problems.

This study was published online, December 1, 2004 on the Proceedings of the National Academy of Sciences. This is an extremely important finding. Most all of us in the health-related professions have long noted the deleterious effects of stress on our patients. This study begins to tell us why. We're not sure how the perception of stress finds its way from the brain to the body's cells, but it appears that it certainly does and with a huge, negative impact. Speeding up aging: REALLY not good. Well, what about the perception of stress?

Remember the old adage, "Beauty is in the eye of the beholder?" Well, of course, that is a true statement. But it goes further than that. Virtually all of human experience is perceived in the eye of the beholder. We all have our own perception of the world and interpret our experiences in a very individualized manner. Therefore, what some people consider stressful, others might not and vice versa. So when you also consider the fact that we all have varying tolerances or thresholds for stress, you can see how complicated this can get. This is one of the reasons why it's impossible to compare human suffering. Consider this: a starving, impoverished, diseased person in an oppressed third world country might be struggling with all of his or her might to survive, yet in your neighborhood an affluent businessman or woman with seemingly everything might attempt to take his or her own life. You cannot compare human suffering. We cannot accurately say that Mary suffers more stress than Jane or Jane suffers more stress than Sue. Look at it this way, for many of us public speaking would be extremely stressful; however, some people thrive doing just such a task. Again, all of human experience is perceived idiosyncratically. Remember this point. It's important.

Life is always in a state of change. That's the one constant or given about life. And it appears to me that human beings just don't care much for change and also don't do particularly well with it. However, our own personal lives are always in a state of change. Life is a process of many unending changes. We must be able to adjust and adapt to the fairly constant change of life and emotionally to accept that life is a process. It is in our best interests to enjoy the process of life. Please don't get caught up in the thinking that says, "I will be happy when...." People can finish that statement with a variety of things including, "I buy my new house, I retire and move to Florida, I find the perfect spouse," etc. If we find ourselves making statements like this, we are not enjoying the process of life. Instead we are trying to find some mythical end-result that is happiness. Unfortunately not only will that not work, but it also serves as a lesson in disappointment. What we are actually doing is keeping happiness at a constant arm's length away. Real happiness is never in obtaining some end result. Remember, the end result to life is death. Let's not rush it. Let's enjoy the process of living.

Another thing that is always changing is the number and kinds of stressors with which we are confronted. It is when the number or intensity of stressors gets unmanageable that we feel "stressed out." If this condition persists, we set ourselves up for physical problems, emotional problems, or both. What I mean is, our body will either break down, or we will become anxious and/ or depressed. Don't forget the connection of stress to obesity, as well as stress and aging. There are several reasons why uncontrolled, chronic stress predisposes a person to obesity and possibly Syndrome X. Stress can undermine your diet, your exercise, your quality of life, and perhaps, the length of your life.

STRESS IN—STRESS OUT

The following diagram presents a simple way to conceptualize stress management. We all have incoming stressors. Stress is inevitable, as I already mentioned. Hopefully, we all have some outlets for stress. As long as our outlets are greater than, or equal to, the incoming stress, we have homeostasis or balance. This balance is crucial because without it we are incapable of managing our stress adequately. Imbalance sets the stage for negative outcomes because when our stressors are greater than our outlets, we are thrown into a state of distress and are inviting physical illness or emotional problems to occur. At the bottom of the diagram you will see some possible *negative* outlets for stress. (Yes, there can be *very* negative outlets for stress!) Sometimes people who are severely stressed develop outlets for stress that are unhealthy. Examples are alcohol abuse, gambling, or excessive overeating. I suspect the use of impulsive, compulsive overeating as a negative outlet for stress is one of the primary reasons why stress is so often associated with obesity. Unfortunately, whatever form they take, these negative outlets circle back around and produce more incoming stressors for us. For instance, after going through a rough time, you realize you've gained twenty pounds, or that you're definitely drinking too much alcohol. In my many years in practice, I have seen many people who realized several months after going through a divorce that they were drinking way too much. Consciously or unconsciously, we try to manage our stress and reduce our emotional pain through whatever means possible.

This is a slippery slope that spirals towards greater distress. That is, our *negative outlets* for stress will always turn around and bite us on the butt.

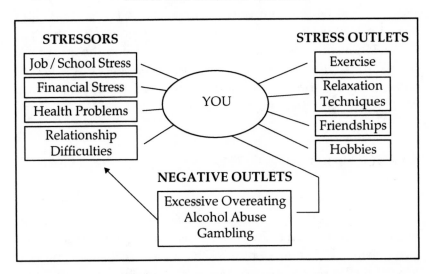

STRESS MANAGEMENT DIAGRAM

Our stressors may stay relatively stable over time, but they are also subject to change rapidly. When increased stress occurs, my first advice to people is to "turn up the outlets." In order to maintain balance, we must find ways to channel that stress out as rapidly as possible. That means spending more time with positive relationships, increasing the amount of play you engage in, increasing your practice of relaxation measures or increasing your exercise. Certainly, there are other outlets besides those listed, but the main thing is to find something positive in your life that you can "turn up." Sometimes we are very fortunate and can actually avoid or terminate some kind of particular stress. However, many times we will simply have to find more effective ways to manage it. I think one of the important things as we go through life is to constantly be looking for potential and seeking new stress outlets. Of course these need to always be *positive* outlets. These, too, are in the eye of the beholder. It's only important that these be positive and serve YOU well as a way to relieve stress. These choices will vary widely from one individual to the next. I know one gentleman who finds a great deal of relief and pleasure from buying old pickup trucks, fixing them up some and selling them later. This works well for him as a stress outlet (I think it may have the opposite effect on his wife!). I know a delightful young woman who, when confronted with increased stress, calls her sister and shares her burden and feels the emotional support of that relationship. So good outlets for stress are in the eye of the beholder, like the rest of human experience. I encourage you to continually experiment and find all the positive outlets that you can. I assure you that you can't have too many.

STRUCTURED RELAXATION

I think some form of relaxation training is always advantageous. There are many avenues available for structured relaxation training or relaxation techniques. These can be quite formal such as biofeedback training or progressive muscle relaxation training. Mental health professionals often do these techniques, and some practitioners offer guides on meditation. In addition to this there are books and cassette tapes available that practice imagery conditioning and other meditative techniques. Yoga classes have proven to be quite valuable. Yoga tends to induce relaxation as well as being an excellent flexibility routine. Just remember that whatever relaxation technique you use, the relaxation response is a learned response. That is, it is not natural for all of us to know how to deeply and profoundly relax. It is an extremely good investment of your time and energy to learn a relaxation technique. Almost any of the relaxation-based procedures that you will practice will elicit the relaxation response. It does take some practice and a little time, but the relaxation response will come. This is always a good stress outlet.

I routinely provide cassette tapes with a short relaxation exercise on it to my patients, when it appears beneficial. They are only about fifteen minutes in length, and on the tape I ask them to focus on the muscles in their body, some positive imagery and sensations, and I include a short breathing exercise. I ask them to listen to the tape one time a day. That is only a fifteen-minute block of time where the only thing that is important for them to do is *relax*. That's really a pretty good deal. Relaxation is physical (relaxing the muscles) and mental (relaxing the mind). The relaxation exercise is aimed toward both of those goals. But relaxation, too, is in the eye of the beholder. Experiment with some different relaxation techniques to find the one that works best for you. Some people definitely respond best to very concrete evidence of relaxation that occurs with biofeedback training. Some people are better hypnotic subjects and do well with hypnosis or imagery-conditioning approaches. I think it is important to schedule fifteen to twenty minutes a day for some form of relaxation training. Certainly, this is one readily available stress outlet for you. The more time you spend in practice, the better you will become.

Okay, this next sentence is really going to shock you. *Life is sometimes difficult*. There, I said it. Surprised? I don't think so. Yes, life can be exceedingly difficult at times. Many times, often beginning in childhood, we are lulled into the perception that once we are an adult, life will be a continuous, beautiful experience. Wrong. In fact, I can personally guarantee you that, at some point, life will be exceedingly difficult. Life is not a continuous, beautiful experience. I think that most of us know this, at least intellectually. Unfortunately, sometimes our intellectual understanding of this statement does not translate into a good emotional understanding of the statement. That is, we may intellectually *know* that "life is difficult," but still, when difficulties arise, we react emotionally with tremendous disappointment and surprise. So you see, emotionally or unconsciously, we are still reacting as if we expect life to be pretty easy. However, life is what it is. It has the potential for tremendous joy and also for tremendous pain. I think it is exceedingly important, therefore, to understand, on an emotional level, that life will sometimes be quite difficult or painful. A good emotional understanding will at least partially prepare you for those times.

So, during times of difficulty, what should you do? Being a male myself, I know exactly what us guys would do. We have two possible options available. One, we can stick our head in the sand and pretend everything is okay. (This is a very popular response!) The only other option we have is to become angry and express our anger in an unproductive, destructive way. There, those are our possibilities. Okay, I'm just kidding, there are other responses that are more appropriate and we need to find them.

TAKING ACTION

As I was alluding to, when those difficult experiences happen, it's a really bad time to pull the covers over your head and do nothing. These are times when you need to "turn up your stress outlets" and do something. You need to develop and use some basic problem-solving skills. When confronted with a particular problem or difficulty in life, generate your options. Make a list of things that you could do. Evaluate those options, and try to determine the consequences of each of them. Take the very best option, and go with it. If it doesn't work, try again. You see, I have a strong bias towards action over inaction. Try to remember to generate the very best options that you can and evaluate them carefully. Pick the very best avenue and proceed. As you continue to develop a more "pro-active" stance, your problem solving skills will improve, and you will be making better decisions. You will find that you are better able to generate a "menu" of possible options. Also, you will find that you are better able to predict the consequences of each of those actions and therefore you will have a better idea of what to do. Taking action makes you an active variable in your life and in a way empowers you. You can become a participant, rather than just a passive "punching bag" for the stressors that impinge upon you. I know it's trial and error, but much of life itself is trial and error. Making decisions and suffering the consequences of those decisions provide fertile earth for something very important: your psychological growth. Living with the consequences of our decisions is an important avenue for learning.

SELF-EFFICACY

Yes, taking action helps manage stress. Psychologists have also written about a concept that has a positive affect on stress and life in general. Sometimes it is called "Sense of control." Sometimes it is called "Self-efficacy." It is often referred to as "Mastery." What self-efficacy, or mastery, means is the feeling, or belief, that you have some control over your destiny and that you are not powerless. You are the major player in the game, and you have some real impact on your life. After all, whose life is it anyway? This is your life, and you are in charge of it. This is not only linked to psychological well-being but also to health, resistance to disease, and longevity. Taking a proactive stance does, in fact, increase your control, and this alone seems to have a beneficial effect in managing stress. In fact, this is one of the most powerful factors in terms of how well we fare in the management of stress. *I cannot overstate how important it is to perceive that you have some control over your life.* Otherwise, we would feel like victims of fate. That sounds like a very bad place to be. Assuming a lack of control over your life invites you to feel powerless and puts you in a very vulnerable, depressing, and depressive life style. It is vitally important that we always have some areas of our life in which we feel control. The more proactive we are, the more control we have.

As an example, throughout most of my career, I have worked quite hard. Many weeks I have worked in excess of 55–60 hours. That would seem like excessive job stress. However, since I am self-employed, I know that I can leave my office anytime I want and have my staff reschedule my clients. Now, I never do this (well, hardly ever), but I know that I *could* do this. It is that sensation of control that, in fact, renders my job fairly stress-free. Basically, control of your life—good; no control—bad. I know there are limits to our control, but we need to seek empowerment. No one wants to feel powerless. Being proactive delivers more power.

SELF-ESTEEM

Another important quality is self-esteem, which is related to self-efficacy or mastery. Self-esteem or good self-confidence is a tremendous asset. It increases our ability to handle stress and it strengthens us against depression. If I had a magic wand and could only use it one time with each one of my clients, this is probably what I would give them. Increasing self-esteem, like so much in life, is an ongoing process. We are constantly challenged to feel good about ourselves. It seems to be a natural human characteristic to tend to believe in the negative about ourselves rather than the positive. Most people are in touch with their weaknesses, more than their strengths. I think that very few people see themselves accurately. Most of us are so self-critical that we see ourselves in a diminished light. I think we fight our little battles most of our lives in order to feel more adequate. It just seems so hard sometimes to shake off our fears and insecurities.

Once, for example, many years ago, I gave a luncheon speech on stress management to about 100 people. After my thirty- or forty-minute presentation on the principles of stress management, I was able to visit with the members of the audience. Many, many people shook my hand and told me how much they enjoyed my talk. However, one person told me that he did not agree with my presentation and that I had some things all wrong. That night, when I was trying to go to sleep, what comment do you think I was thinking about? Do you think I was thinking of the eighty or so positive responses to my speech? No. I was thinking of the one individual who was critical. Again, this seems to be human nature. We latch onto any of the negative feedback that we get, even if it's in the vast minority. It would be very helpful if we were more mindful of the positive feedback that we get. However, much of the time we seem to ignore it. What a shame. Think about that the next time someone gives you a compliment. A compliment is a gift. When you are given a gift, it is good etiquette to accept that gift graciously. Think about it.

In many ways, good self-esteem is a process of loving yourself. It is very important to get in touch with those positive, healthy aspects of yourself and truly experience them. Give yourself some credit. It is not selfish or evil or wrong for you to care for yourself. Not at all. In fact, it's an exceedingly beautiful thing to love and care for yourself. It is really true what some of the older scholars have said, "You have to love yourself before you are able to have the maximum amount to give others."

Take a moment and think about how you treat some object that you own that you really truly value. Chances are that you take exceedingly good care of it. I bet you make sure that you keep it clean, in proper running order, and well maintained. *I want you to value you yourself that much.* I want you to embrace your importance and love yourself so much that you care for yourself enthusiastically. I want you to value yourself so much that you properly maintain and take care of yourself on all levels. You are valuable enough to keep your weight in a normal range. It's okay to care how you look and how you feel. You are worth keeping yourself strong, fit, and active. It's okay for you to play, have fun, and experience joy. Think about it. Give yourself some love. Give yourself a lot of love.

WHAT ARE YOU THINKING?

One important thing you are going to have to do is watch out for your thinking. Yes, by golly, your thinking. This too can turn around and become self-defeating. That's right, you have to watch the content of your thoughts. We all have these ongoing, almost automatic thoughts all the time. They are referred to as self-statements—that is, something that we are telling ourselves in our own head. As mentioned, many of these thoughts tend to become automatic over the years, especially those thoughts that relate to how we are evaluating ourselves. Remember, we tend to have a proneness to evaluate ourselves negatively (I mentioned that before, were you paying attention?). Therefore, many of us walk around with a high number of negative self-statements, and these can certainly make us feel bad. There is a huge array of possibilities for negative self-statements. The following are a few negative self-statements. See if you say any of these. If not, try to figure out what your negative self-statements are.

- I can't do anything right.
- I am not very smart.
- Nobody seems to like me.
- I am too old, fat, ugly, or whatever.
- I am never going to feel good.
- I can't stand it.
- Nothing good ever happens to me.

Just imagine if you are saying these kinds of things to yourself; **how would you expect to feel!?** You are going to feel bad. No question about it, if you have much of this garbage going on upstairs, you're going to be feeling bad. Try to identify those negative self-statements and stop them. If you can't stop them, you are going to have to at least slow them down. Try to increase the number of positive self-statements you make. Just as negative self-statements can make you feel bad, positive self-statements can make you feel good. (Who knew!) Try practicing some positive self-statements such as these:

- I can do it.
- I am as competent as anyone else.
- I can have good friends by being a good friend.
- I am going to stay focused on the task at hand.
- My life is good.
- I am as well off as most other people.
- I try to do the "right" thing.
- I have many things to be thankful for.

Try this the next time you are having a "bad day": stop for a moment and try to evaluate what you have been thinking. Nine times out of ten, you've been ambushing yourself with negative self-statements. With this awareness, you can begin to change. Stay conscious of this. If necessary, and it most often is, post written positive self-statements on your bathroom mirror and on the computer monitor that you work on at the office. Basically, write them down and place them anywhere that you are usually forced to look throughout the day. Stay aware and watch what you are thinking. Many times we think that our negative emotions produce negative thinking. That can sometimes be true. However, many times our negative thinking produces negative emotions. As mentioned, our positive thoughts can promote positive emotions. The bottom line here is that thought often precedes emotion. Read that again out loud. *Thought often precedes emotion.* Let's try to manage those thoughts much better. If you do, you'll probably feel better.

BEHAVE!

Okay, *thinking* certainly does play a major role in our self-perception and how we feel, but so does *behavior*. Almost every time I leave my Mom after a visit, she says, "Behave." She has been saying that for most of my life (and believe me, she needed to). But what does she mean by that? Well, as a psychologist I am perfectly aware that I am always "behaving." What she means though is to act in a manner that is self-enhancing and not self-defeating. It is actually very good advice. If we manage our behavior so that we are, in fact, behaving in ways we are proud of, it is likely to increase our self-esteem. Sometimes I ask clients to give me a short list of attributes that they admire in others. It could be such things as kindness, generosity, humor, purpose, and so forth. I then ask them to try to "practice" these behaviors in their day-to-day life. If they will practice those attitudes that they deem positive, they have a pretty good chance of developing more positive feelings about themselves. Of course, the inverse is also true. If you find yourself engaged in behaviors that you are ashamed of, it can damage your self-esteem.

You see, we all tend to have certain basic beliefs that we live by, and these may be conscious or unconscious. This is called a *belief system*. Whether conscious or unconscious, it plays a powerful role. If our behavior runs contrary to our belief system, we then create a *behavior-belief discrepancy* that leads to conflict and emotional pain. For example, if you believe lying is wrong, yet you find yourself engaging in it, this could have a negative effect on your self-esteem. So, it is a good idea to determine what your basic belief systems are, especially in terms of personal code of conduct or ethics and to try to keep your behavior in line with your belief system. It is much easier to love yourself when you don't create behavior-belief discrepancies. It's kind of like this: if you become like someone you admire in terms of conduct, ethics and so on, then you tend to begin to admire yourself. That is a very good thing. You see what I mean? Admire yourself, love yourself, and value yourself. If all that were true, you would probably take care of yourself. You might even consider a nutritious diet and a well-planned exercise routine!

LOVE YOURSELF AND PASS IT ON

If you love yourself, you should give yourself some gifts. What kind of gifts? Anything that can enhance your joy and sense of peace in your life would work. Perhaps the gift of a little more time; maybe it would be nice to have thirty minutes when you get home from work to just sit in your chair and read the paper, relax, or whatever. Maybe it would be nice to give yourself an outing from time to time. How about getting a massage? How about taking a vacation? Too many people think that showing themselves a kindness is "selfish." I do not, and I do not think you should either. I think that it is self-enhancing. I believe that when you give yourself gifts, which promote your own happiness and well-being, you are better prepared to give back to others. When we see to it that our own needs are met, then we are much more able to meet the needs of others. For example, if I am not taking good care of myself and I am unhappy, I am probably not as good a friend, son, husband, father, or therapist as I could be. When I am happy and taking care of myself, I, indeed, am a better friend, son, husband, father, therapist and so on. You see, even in terms of the care you give others, you have to make your own needs a priority. To be a caregiver, you must start with yourself. It is only then that you have the power it takes to give maximally back to others.

Just as accepting yourself as important, it is also important how you accept others. Very often, important people in our lives will do certain things that cause us pain and disappointment. We have to remember to accept others, not as we wish them to be, but as they actually are. I think very often we go through little "power struggles" with relationships in our life, trying to make them ideal for us. We would be far better served if we really understood the other person and accepted them as they are. Again too often, we look at relationships in terms of how we wish them to be, rather than how they really are. That leads me right to the next topic.

BASIC "DUCK" PSYCHOLOGY

It's like I tell my clients, "If it looks like a duck, walks like a duck, and swims like a duck, it indeed is probably a duck." Should we expect it to soar like an eagle? No. Should we expect it to hoot like an owl? No. Should we expect it to crawl on its belly like a snake? No. Why? **BECAUSE IT'S A DUCK!** (Are you listening?) That is all it is, and that is all it will be. And there is nothing wrong with it being a duck. A duck is beautiful. And let's face it; the world would not be such a beautiful place without ducks. Therefore, if someone in your life has a consistent way of behaving that annoys you or hurts your feelings, you probably need to get over it. If a family member has not given you the response you wanted in forty years, then they are probably not going to give it to you. Just like a duck, they are what they are. They are beautiful and you love them anyway. Again, we would not expect a duck to soar like an eagle or to hoot like an owl, so don't expect this person in your life to behave in a manner that you find desirable. Remember, we have to love and accept others for the way they are, not how we wish them to be. Very often, it is not other people who directly disappoint us. It is *our expectations* of other people that, more directly, disappoint us. Our expectations are part of our "self." They are a part of our personal belief system. The other people in our lives are not responsible for or subject to our expectations. Those are our responsibilities. It is far more likely that we will be able to change our expectations of others, rather than have them change themselves to meet our expectations. Getting back to our analogy, don't be surprised when a duck quacks! Remember, it's what a duck does. We should indeed expect a duck to quack. Love your ducks anyway. Don't let them throw you off balance.

Stress management is all about balance. Balancing our stress outlets so that they are at least equal to our stressors. Self-statements have to be balanced in order that we have at least as many positives as we have negatives. This helps us hang on to our self-esteem and gives us some feeling of control in our life. We also have to keep our behavior-belief systems balanced so as to not create conflict. Keep your balance. Keep healthy.

CHAPTER 14

Pursuit of Happiness

IT'S TRUE; it's very difficult sometimes to break psychological inertia. Depression often yields to hopelessness and it is near impossible to exercise and eat correctly when you feel hopeless. Let's face it, when we feel this way exercise and diet don't even matter. In fact, when we feel like this, not much at all does matter. This is that negative psychological inertia where "objects at rest tend to remain at rest." The relationship between the physical and the emotional is crystal clear. Hopelessness does not have just emotional ramifications but physical ones as well. Despair and depression are also correlated with physical illness, poor response to surgery or other treatment, and even earlier death. Exercise can help. If the depressed patient can "make" him or herself exercise, their depression will improve, but it is just so hard to act that most of the time depressed individuals just don't. Sometimes the first task is to "feel better" before exercising and healthy dieting can begin. When it does begin, this contributes to a positive or healthy cycle. That is, the better you feel, the more you will exercise and watch your nutrition, and the more you exercise and eat well, the better you feel. Each promotes the other. Now we have a new kind of inertia, a positive one where "objects in motion remain in motion." In this condition much personal change and growth can occur. First, you have to feel good. Regardless of what it takes, this is a priority. We have become "an object in motion."

From time to time, in my career, I have had the opportunity to be invited to speak to various groups. They were usually fairly small groups, but sometimes they were quite large and the topics would vary quite a bit. Sometimes I would be asked to speak about stress management. Other times I would be asked to speak on dealing with trauma. Very often, during the question and answer segment after the talk, I would ask several of the individuals, "What do you want most?" Invariably, the most common answer was, "I want to be happy." Of course; who doesn't? Well, all right then, how do we do that? What does it mean to be happy? Certainly, this is something that we all want. We probably spend most of our energies chasing this desirable condition, whether we know it or not. The daunting question appears to be, "How do we get it? What must we do to be happy?" We can see people living their lives, going in all directions, trying to obtain this elusive emotional position. I have spent most of my rather long career observing people and interacting with people in regard to the pursuit of their happiness, as well as being in the hunt myself. In this chapter, we'll take a look at a few things that probably do make you happy, and discuss a few things that I think probably will not.

WHAT'S MONEY GOT TO DO WITH IT?

"I don't care too much for money, money can't buy me love." So goes the old rock and roll song. So how about it? What do you think?

My dad has lived a long life. In his life he has gained, what I consider, much wisdom. He used to ask me, "Do you want to feel richer?" Of course, the answer was invariably, "Yes!" (Who wouldn't?) Then he would say, "Well, then want a lot less." Good point. Wanting what you don't have can sure make you feel poor. It would serve us better if we wanted and valued what we have, instead of putting too much energy into desiring what we do not have. Buddha said, "Life is suffering." We have already arrived at the conclusion that life is difficult. I can see the similarity, can't you? Buddha went on to say that most suffering comes from cravings, that is, wanting what we don't have.

The Bible says that the love of money is the root of all evil. It also says that coveting that which is not yours is self-defeating. This particular wisdom is ancient. I think there is something to it, don't you? Wanting what you don't have can certainly contribute to emotional pain.

How about money? Can it make you happy? I think the relationship between money and happiness is kind of strange. You see, frankly, the lack of money can pretty well make you unhappy. Yes, if you don't have enough money to meet the monthly obligations you have, and you are struggling and suffering, certainly that feels stressful. For many of us, financial stress or worrying about money is a constant stressor in our lives. Balancing our income against our expenditures demands a lot of attention and sometimes sacrifices. However, it has been my experience that having considerably more money, after you meet those basic necessities, does very little to improve the *quality* of your life. That is, it doesn't make you happier. Acquiring and spending money is just a part of life, not the cornerstone of our happiness. I have just seen too many people in my practice over the last twenty-six years who had plenty of money, yet were miserable. Now, don't get me wrong. There is nothing wrong with money. I am not saying that. Having money is fine. Certainly, I want you to have enough money. I am simply saying that you cannot rely on money as the key to lasting happiness. It's like not being able to see the forest for the trees. Too many people spend all their time chasing around for more and more money only to continue to have disappointing lives. Do you know anyone like this?

HOW ABOUT STUFF?

Can a lot of cool stuff make you happy? I have seen many people save and save for their "dream house." They just know they will really be happy when they get the house of their dreams. Unfortunately, I have often seen them move into that dream house only to find them divorcing around twelve to eighteen months later. The house just didn't work for "happy," folks. Have you ever done this? Have you ever saved for that special car that you really, really wanted? When you got it, it was a great feeling. You got so excited every time you walked across the parking lot to it or pulled it out of your garage in the morning. After about a year … it was just a car. Yep, just a car. Just plain old transportation. No, I don't think stuff makes you happy either. (My Harley might be an exception here!) Again, don't get me wrong. Just like money, there is nothing wrong with having some "stuff." It's great to have things that you really like. I think it's far better to have a few things that are really important to you rather than a lot of things that are fairly meaningless. I want you to have the house that you like, car that you like, clothes that you like, and so on. Just don't look for it to give you a life that is a continuous, beautiful experience.

In fact, most of our material possessions provide us with a brief period of excitement. It seems like the "newness" of many things is the best part. Of course, some things we continue to enjoy for years and years. These are those things that do mean a lot to us, and while we enjoy having them, they do not produce a pervasive sense of happiness. We're going to have to look someplace else for that.

You know, it's a funny thing about stuff. It seems, in terms of our lifespan, we spend our 20s and 30s, and sometimes part of our 40s, accumulating stuff. Then, when we reach our 50s and 60s, we start trying to give our stuff away. It always seems like less is more by that point in life. By then you probably have begun to figure out what the key to happiness really is. It is not money (although there is nothing wrong with that) and it is not a lot of cool stuff (although there is nothing wrong with that either). You see, it's not all about getting what you want. It's about wanting what you have!

RELATIONSHIPS

Well then, what does make you happy? I know the answer and I am going to tell you. It's relationships. The quality and quantity of the relationships in our lives is vital to determining our happiness. A healthy and thriving primary, or spousal, relationship is extremely important in overall happiness. Important I said, not sufficient. Sometimes when we are young, we believe that a healthy, primary relationship is the key to happiness. Well, it is one of the keys because it has the capacity to bring us so much joy. A thriving and dynamic primary relationship is, indeed, wonderful. But remember, no one person is going to be able to meet all of your emotional needs. Besides, the things that can give us the most joy can also bring us the most pain. Developing the skills and understanding to nurture and maintain a thriving primary relationship is no easy task. These relationships require a tremendous amount of work and commitment but offer so much in return. But again, no single relationship, regardless of how good it is, can meet all of our emotional needs. Therefore, it is not sufficient, in and of itself, for enduring, pervasive happiness.

Good relationships with our family members are very important. This is especially true for those very close to us, such as our parents and our children. They are vital to our personal happiness. Yes, I know, sometimes a member of our family will emotionally injure us or disappoint us in some way, but recovering and repairing is extremely important. Our family is a potentially enormous source of emotional strength. I am sure our need for strong family relationships predates recorded history. Remember Paleolithic Bob? Without family, Bob and all those like him would not have survived. They needed each other in many very concrete ways. Mankind has survived because we are social creatures. That is, our interconnectedness and inter-reliance gave us collective strength, which reinforced our evolutionary success. Staying emotionally connected to family is very important. Remember family is our first "tribe" or "clan."

Good friends are absolutely wonderful, too. In our modern society, many times our good friends are actually related to as family. Because we tend to be rather mobile and many times suddenly work in areas that are rather remote from our biological family, our friends provide emotional support just as family members do. Perhaps you don't have to have a huge number of friends—I am biased to think quality is over quantity here. Having one or two people with whom you can be completely open, trust, and rely on is a tremendous source of emotional strength. Friendships are often extremely durable. By that I mean a good friendship will very often last a lifetime and that makes it rare and precious. You see, we derive most of our real happiness and satisfaction with life from positive relationships with others. Now, self-reliance is a good thing. Just like self-efficacy and self-confidence, it helps us manage the stress of life. However, without some good, positive friendships in our life, our existence would be quite empty.

As you can see, there are many types of relationships (parent, child, spousal, friend) that we experience in life. All are important in terms of developing and maintaining our *emotional support network*. Each type of relationship contributes in terms of being a source of emotional strength that helps us weather the stressors of life. It is our responsibility to develop and maintain those relationships. Therefore, we have to be aware of how we are relating, both verbally and non-verbally, in order to avoid potential trouble. Thus, our interpersonal skills are of utmost value. It is important that we learn to practice positive traits such as kindness, patience, respect and so on. These are some of the skills necessary to develop and maintain healthy relationships. For instance, if we want good friends, we have to be a good friend, in order to have those friendships work. If we want positive family relationships, we have to behave in a positive manner towards those family members. Oh, of course, in any close relationship, there will be some conflicts that arise from time to time. The real strength of a relationship is knowing that you can disagree about something today, but it will not jeopardize the future endurance of your relationship. We need to feel like we are in a network of relationships that involve mutual love and respect in order for us to really feel okay—happy. ***Relationships are to us emotionally, what food is to us physically.*** Without them we would starve. We could not successfully live. We absolutely have to have them. Social isolation nearly always yields depression and illness. As I mentioned earlier, Dr. Dean Ornish, in his book, *Love and Survival*, dramatically illustrates that feeling emotionally connected to others increases our chance of recovery from illness and injury. That's why I know we desperately need these relationships. Without them we die, one way or the other. Just like Paleolithic Bob, relationships help us survive.

When I have the occasion to talk with terminally ill patients, I always learn a great deal. It is a distinct privilege to have this opportunity. It helps to clarify what is important in life and what is not. For instance, I have never had a terminally ill patient say, "Gee, Dr. Ken, I wish I had worked more Saturdays." I have never had a terminally ill patient say, "I wish I had made more money," or "I wish I had been a little meaner to others." What they do talk about, and smile about, are their experiences in relationships with the people whom they have loved. In the final analysis, this is one of the most important things. To love and be loved is the centerpiece of human existence and happiness. Relationships, like life, are always in a process of being. Remember, change is the constant in life, and relationships are not immune to this. They require maintenance through effort and patience. And, like exercise, the dividends are usually proportionate to the investment. The more we put into them (even though at times it can be a little painful), the more we reap in rewards. Remember, what food is to us physically, relationships are to us emotionally. We absolutely have to have them.

Why not start at the top and consider your relationship with your God and then develop a strategy for enhancing it. That's right. There is plenty of evidence that a belief in a higher power is, in many cases, linked to human happiness. Many people derive a huge sense of support or strength from their religious belief system. It's like plugging in to a power source and from that place of strength, investing in the other relationships in your world. Feeling connected to something larger than ourselves can help us find peace.

Focus then on family, friends, associates, and so on, working to increase the quality of these relationships, and feel your emotional support system grow. How do you work on these? Kindness works wonders. Learn to help set the emotional tone through good eye contact and pleasant facial expression (maybe smile a bit more) when greeting others. Learn to communicate better by listening better and expressing yourself more clearly. Demonstrate respect by not interrupting when others are speaking. Be aware of your voice tone and volume. Notice your delivery. Sometimes it really is not what you say, but how you say it. Think about it—there are many ways to enhance these relationships.

WORK AND PLAY

Isn't it true?—there's so much to do and so little time. What should we do with our time? My grandpa said, "If you want to be happy, work eight hours a day, play eight hours a day, and sleep eight hours a day." My grandpa was a very, very smart man.

One of the things that I have learned in my career is that people who work are generally happier than people who don't. Now don't get me wrong here; I am not talking about people who just hold down a job. Homemakers and mothers have a tremendous job to do. Perhaps their job is the most important. In all the animal kingdom, raising healthy offspring to adulthood appears to be the primary job or purpose. That's why you and I are here today, the biological imperative to reproduce and raise successful offspring. Raising children is a tremendous job and responsibility. It's also one of the most difficult and demanding jobs I can think of.

But work is still work, right? Oh sure, regardless of what kind of job we have, we all complain about it and gripe about it some, but still, it seems to be an important player in the happiness game. Why? Basically, we all need some reason to get up in the morning. We need some sense of meaning or purpose in our life. Also, we have a terrible dilemma structuring our own time. You know, you're born at point A and you die at point Z. So how do you fill out the area in between? I think this is one of the most puzzling problems of the human experience. "This is my life and the minutes are ticking past. What do I want to do with it?" When you have a job, it does that for you, in large measure. You know where you are going to be at 8:00 Monday morning and about what time you will be getting off and coming home. It keeps us focused on a task, which is an excellent diversion from other stressors in our life. Like I said, structuring our time is an important task in our life. Work helps.

Of course, I think it is really important to find the right type of work for you. Finding a job that brings you some satisfaction is wonderful. Finding a job that you're passionate about is even better. We really need things to feel passionate about. Sometimes we need to work on our attitude about the job. I mean, if it's not your "dream job" you still can look at the positives that are there. Perhaps it can be a vehicle for making new friends or offer the chance to learn new skills. Find the very best aspects of the job and maximize them. Our job needs to be important to us because it represents a large part of our life.

Sometimes I see individuals who have quit work. Either they have become disabled or simply retired. This change can be a very difficult time. We go from a lifetime of going to work to, all of a sudden, having no job to go to at all. Much of our personal identity is tied up in our job, whether at home or away. When that is taken away, we really lose something. Occasionally, I will suggest to my clients that they consider doing some volunteer work. I usually suggest a local hospital as a place for them to inquire. The results of this have been rather dramatic. They usually get service type, volunteer positions at the hospital. Perhaps they greet people and give out information, or they actually help transport patients to the cafeteria or to some of their diagnostic tests. At any rate, they render a service. I have certainly learned from their experience that serving others is generally very rewarding. My clients come back to me enthused, excited and fulfilled because they have seen and felt themselves be of service to others. Basically, when we serve others, our own cup is also filled. Giving and receiving become one! That's a very beautiful thing about the human spirit; it feels good to help others. This kind of activity actually serves two purposes. It aids in structuring our time as well as giving us a sense of contribution or purpose.

So, if you are working, throw yourself into your job. Focus on it and do a great job at whatever you are doing. Look for and maximize the positives that are there. Find something in your job situation to get excited about. Develop a passion for it. Develop ways to provide a service or kindness to others while performing the duties of your job. You will just feel better. The more you invest, the larger the dividend! Whether in the home or in the office, people who work are happier than people who don't.

That brings me to another issue. Significance. Yes, the notion that we are significant and that we all matter somehow in the great scheme of things. You can see how this fits in with the concept that we all need a sense of purpose and meaning in our lives. I think that we all would like to think that our lives mean something and that the world will somehow be a better place because we were here. Yet, I talk to so many of my clients who complain that they feel insignificant, unimportant, and ordinary. *Ordinary!* I explain to them that, in fact, most of us are "ordinary." I don't see anything really wrong with ordinary. Often they will look back at me and say something like, "But you've made something of your life." I generally respond, "Yep, I've experienced some accomplishments and made many mistakes. I guess that is 'something,' just like you." You see, most of us (the vast majority of us) are ordinary. No, we won't win a Nobel Prize or discover a cure for cancer because, by golly, we are ordinary. But you know what, we ordinary people can plant a tree, pick up a piece of litter, put out a bird feeder, adopt an unwanted pet, be thoughtful of the elderly, respect the disabled and disadvantaged, and perform innumerable other acts that make a difference. In fact, it's impossible to measure how big of a difference it can make. You see, even "ordinary people" can leave the world a far better place because they have been here. Ordinary and insignificant do not mean the same thing. We can obtain significance through work and non-work activities. We can all be significant.

All work and no play? Of course not! I am encouraging you to play. I don't care how old you are—you need to play. We don't quit playing because we get old. We get old because we quit playing. Remember that I said that beauty is in the eye of the beholder? Remember, also, I said that all of human experience is really in the eye of the beholder? Therefore, what is play for me may not be play for you. You will have to discover those things that provide play for you and that you can become passionate about. One of the ways that I play is to ride my motorcycle. Some of you would find that to be boring and others of you would find that to be terrifying. You see, we all perceive experiences in our own way. So, I want you to find out what will work for you.

Now that you have already gotten yourself in good shape through your exercise and diet program, you may want to engage in some sports for play. Again, regardless of age, sports can be invigorating. If you are over 40, you could qualify to participate in Master's Track and Field. Pick an event and start training and start playing. If you are over 50, you can train for the Senior Olympics. Here, there are even more events to choose from, and surely some of those would be fun for you. What about softball? Have you played? It could be fun. How about bowling, fishing, hunting, tennis, badminton, or whatever? Use some experimentation and, through trial and error, find some activities that are "fun" for you and keep them up. Learn to play bridge, card games, and board games. These constitute play also. Unfortunately, play becomes a lost art as we age. Let's reclaim it. Remember, we are talking about rejuvenation.

Here's an idea for you—take up something new. From time to time in a person's life, I think it can be fun and exciting to learn something completely new. Even better, become an "expert" in some novel field. Buy some books on a new subject and study. The prospects appear infinite. Take a photography class. Take a computer class. Take up watercolor. Act in a local play. Become competent at some new skill and play. The results are amazing!

There is fairly recent evidence that staying actively involved in social and mentally challenging leisure activities is beneficial in terms of retaining memory skills. In the *Journal of Epidemiology and Community Health* an article reported that middle-aged adults who were passionate about their social and leisure time activities scored higher on tests of memory, vocabulary, and math than those who were no longer participating in the activities that they once enjoyed. You see, it is vital to continue to challenge ourselves throughout our lifetime. Remember what "training stimulus" was when discussing exercise? It is necessary in order for our body to respond positively to the exercise experience. The same concept also applies in this arena. We have to challenge ourselves socially, psychologically, and mentally in order to stay sharp and dynamic.

PRACTICE SOME HUMOR

Humor is another one of those attitudinal variables that just make life more fun. Laughter appears to have some positive effects even on the biochemical level. I think around three "belly laughs" a day promotes the release of endorphins, the body's own antidepressant, and that has got to be good for you. This is some strong evidence that humor is healthy for our mood and can be a powerful and excellent outlet for our ability to manage stress. Look for reasons to laugh. Listen to jokes and funny stories. Read the comics. Seek out comedies at the movie theater. Seek out relationships with people who make you laugh. I, personally, know some really funny people. These types of people are really good for us. Some of my friends are absolutely hysterical and I always feel better after I have been around them. Also learn to laugh at yourself. This is a critically important issue. (I think we tend to take ourselves too seriously.) We are much more lenient on others than we are on ourselves. When you make mistakes, learn to laugh. In fact, many of the most difficult situations in life occur because we take ourselves so seriously that we lose the ability to find humor in what we do. Try to lighten up. If you look for the humor, you will very likely find it. Really, we're all pretty funny. I mean really, as a species, we're funny. People-watch a little more, and I think you'll see what I mean.

Is the evening news always bad? Skip it. You don't have to watch the news every day. If it tends to cause you concern or worry, skip it. Same with the newspaper. If it makes you sad, or concerned, or worried, skip it. We tend to get bombarded by negatives more and more, and these can have a negative effect on our attitude. Every day look for something to smile about. Better yet, laugh out loud, very loud. Never, ever, miss a chance to laugh. Laughter really is a great medicine. Have some daily.

FORGIVENESS

I have a very simple truth for you. Forgiveness is a good thing. Grudges are a bad thing. No question about it. I have witnessed this truth many times. When you hold a grudge, and you are angry with someone, you basically end up punishing yourself. Why would you want to do that? You walk around with all of these negative feelings, feeling bad, feeling angry, and, probably, depressed. Your thoughts are likely exceedingly negative. How do you expect to feel? Let it go. It may seem hard, but work toward it. Forgiveness is also good medicine. It is unimaginably powerful. Humans are imperfect. You're imperfect. I'm imperfect. Everybody is imperfect. Because we are imperfect, we make mistakes. Some of those mistakes hurt others, and other people's mistakes will hurt you. Practice forgiveness. Forgiveness is very healing. Remember, when you can't forgive, you keep being punished over and over again. That's not good for you. Let it go. I cannot over-emphasize how important this is. In a way, it is sort of like service to others. That is, the more we forgive, the more we are healed.

That chip that you carry on your shoulder could be one of your heaviest stressors. As long as you carry it, you continue to exhibit negative thoughts and continue to have negative behavior. Experiment and find what it takes for you to forgive. Talk to a professional counselor or minister if you need to. Whatever it takes. It's that important. Be aware. Be mindful of it. Talk sense to yourself. Practice forgiveness. Oh yes, forgive yourself, too.

In a similar vein, I've learned that it is vitally important to accept the responsibility of our own imperfections or mistakes. We have taken a huge step when we learn to say, "I'm sorry, I made a mistake." When you can accept responsibility for and admit to your own errors, you begin to strip away the guarded, defensive nature that we all seem to have. Those defenses that we carry around like personal armor inhibit our own growth.

Another word about forgiving yourself: we have all done things that we deeply regret. (I know this very well.) We can all look at our past and beat ourselves up over some mistakes we have made again and again. This negative behavior is destructive and has no redeeming qualities. Remember, nobody wakes up and looks around one day and says, "What can I do today that will screw up my life forever?" Of course not! Remember, we all make the best decisions that we can at the time we make them with the information we have at our disposal. Take a moment and read that last sentence again. We are not actively seeking pain and disappointment at all. The problem is, just too much of the time, we don't have adequate information at our disposal. I think every important decision that we make is made on the basis of inadequate information. Let's just accept the fact that really we're all doing the very best that we can. Not near perfect; but the best we can, and always working to improve. We can at least learn something from those past mistakes. Life is always a work in progress.

GETTING OLD?

Don't get anxious about aging. Remember what rejuvenation means. "To be made youthful, again," and I think now you realize this is both physical, mental, and the interaction of the two. Maintain and reclaim those abilities and activities of youth and keep that positive attitude. Keep your life full. There's no reason not to. Aging is natural, but in many ways, getting old is a choice.

I remember when I turned 40, my Mom said, "You're getting too old to keep lifting those weights." Well, this time Mom was wrong. When I turned 50, she said, "You're gonna tear up your back if you keep lifting those weights." Again, she was wrong. Well, not totally. My back is a little "iffy" some days. Just enough to slow me down but not stop me. Don't give yourself permission to miss some important activities or events because you've had a certain birthday. Let me remind you that one of my buddies ran his first complete marathon at the age of 52. Another friend of mine began competitive power lifting at the age of 57. Yet another took up javelin and discus throwing at the age of 48. In short, stubbornly refuse to buy into the old stereotypes. Age really is just a number. The old cliché is really true; *you are as young as you feel.* I'm inviting you to feel very, very young. Try to remember one of my favorite proverbs, "You're only young once, but you can be immature forever." In this regard, I would invite you once again to read an excellent book, *Breaking the Rules of Aging* by Dr. David A. Lipschitz. It is an illuminating work on the aging process, and I strongly recommend it. Every doctor should read it, and anyone over fifty should read it as well. Don't worry about age. Instead, focus on life. Live life to the fullest. Seek joy and tranquility. Seek play and activity. Take your life back. Eat correctly, exercise intelligently, and embrace life to the fullest. Try not to miss a thing and have as few regrets as possible.

CHAPTER 15

Putting It All Together

ATTITUDE AND HEALTH BEHAVIOR

YOU SEE IT CAN WORK EITHER WAY. Attitude sometimes precedes behavior. By that I mean, you can get mentally "pumped up" and enthusiastically embark on self-improvement. With the right attitude, beginning to eat healthier and exercise intelligently can come fairly easily. If your attitude is "super charged," you can use diet and exercise to transform your body dramatically and rather quickly. This change in your body can serve in "pumping up" your attitude even more. It becomes a very positive and healthy cycle.

However, sometimes behavior precedes attitude. By that I mean that sometimes we must take action in order to affect a change in our attitude or emotions. For instance, if you are able to push yourself to go to the gym and start exercising, and begin to practice some better dietary habits, you may soon find that your attitude is dramatically improved and your motivation is high. Even if you are somewhat down or depressed prior to beginning your lifestyle change, you will find that your mood is somewhat transformed through your behavior. In each of these scenarios, one side supports the other. A more active and healthy lifestyle can promote better mood and self-esteem. Conversely, better mood and self-esteem can help fuel a more active and healthy lifestyle. That's what I mean when I say it can work either way.

Now, I mentioned earlier that if you have a significant form of depression, embarking on a self-improvement program may be nearly impossible. I do believe that if you have a clinically significant depression, the first place to start is with your primary care physician and perhaps a mental health referral. If you do have a significant depression, there are a variety of medications that have proven to be very effective in treatment of these disorders. Psychotherapy, in combination with medication, is an even better choice. So if you have a clinically significant mood disorder, you may best be served by beginning to get medical and psychological help first. After receiving such help, you will find that you are much better able to embark upon the kind of self-improvement and lifestyle changes delineated in this book. Make no mistake about it, I believe that exercise can be a potent adjunct to the treatment of anxiety and depression and I continually recommend it. While it can be a powerful assistant, it does not replace prudent psychological/medical care.

REVISITING INERTIA

Let's revisit our psychological model of inertia once again. One of the common analogies that physical science teachers use to instruct us in the law of inertia is the analogy of a stalled automobile. What they tell us is that it takes a great deal of energy to push the automobile in order to get it rolling. Once it is rolling, it takes less energy for it to continue rolling. This is inertia. Remember, objects at rest tend to remain at rest, and objects in motion tend to remain in motion. Therefore, it may take a bit of "push" to begin any self-enhancing lifestyle program. But remember, once you begin to "roll" a little, progress becomes more rapid. When it comes to diet, maybe you need to begin by just having a salad for one meal of the day. Or perhaps, like that patient I discussed earlier, you just need to eat three pieces of fruit a day and leave off the soft drinks. You can start at any place that you are able. Any positive change does represent a push toward achieving a break in your stationary inertia. As you become an object in motion, it is much easier to maintain your momentum. In fact, it is easier to increase your momentum.

DIETS

Remember that structured, restrictive diets don't work. Oh sure, they can give you some short-term results. There have been a plethora of diets in the past fifteen or twenty years that have been able to do that. However, if you look at long-term, permanent weight control, you are looking at something very different. Permanent weight control requires a change in lifestyle. You are looking at including into your diet healthy and nutritious foods and excluding unhealthy, calorie dense foods. One of your primary challenges is to discover those healthy foods that you enjoy eating and make them part of your regular diet. It is also important that you continue to experiment and constantly try to expand the menu of these healthy foods that you can include in your diet. Conversely, it is important to find the unhealthy foods that you can begin to exclude from your diet without feeling deprived. If you continue to experiment with these concepts, I promise that over time you will find that this is no longer a "diet"; instead it is the way that you normally eat. No longer will there be a sense of deprivation or sacrifice. It is not so much adhering to a diet, as it is a change in lifestyle. It is basically a lifestyle change that involves better, more intelligent nutrition.

EXERCISE

Likewise, when it comes to exercise, you are once again trying to break your inertia. If in fact you are an "object at rest," it will take quite a push to get you rolling. However, once you begin rolling, it will be easier and easier to maintain your momentum. In that regard, I urge you to begin with wherever you are and increase your activity level to some extent. Maybe all that you can do is a five-minute walk. If that is so, fine. You have to begin somewhere. A five-minute walk this week can be a seven-minute walk next week and a ten-minute walk in a few weeks. Remember that any activity over and beyond what you are used to will in fact be "exercise." Don't forget the training stimulus. Any challenge to your body greater than what it is used to will elicit the positive change in your strength and stamina.

Cardiovascular training is exceedingly important, not just in terms of the quality of your life but perhaps in the quantity of your life as well. Start with wherever you are and try to eventually work up to forty or so minutes a day. Cardiovascular training should be done near daily but at minimum four days a week. I promise that you get dividends returned in accordance with the investment that you make. Cardiovascular training will aid you in burning body fat and give you an excellent stress management outlet. Don't forget the buddy system. As with all types of exercise, success is more easily attained when you exercise with a friend.

Strength training or resistance training can reshape your body. Strength training, with proper diet, can rapidly change your body composition and enhance your appearance. It enables you to feel strong and feeling strong is always good. Strength training and the resulting change in body composition can have a profound effect on body image. Body image can, in fact, have a strong influence on self-esteem. Self-esteem can have a profound influence on mood. As your mood and enthusiasm grow, it is much easier to engage in a high-level exercise program. Remember the interconnectedness of the mind and body. Strength training can be done intelligently two to four times a week. The investment of time is actually minimal, requiring only 20-40 minutes a work out. Again, the physical and psychological benefits are not only significant but also downright amazing.

Flexibility training is another valuable outlet for stress. Flexibility training can easily be accomplished as the "cool down" part of any workout, whether it is cardiovascular, resistance training or both. It only takes a few minutes to do the basic stretching exercises and the payoff is excellent. Flexibility does not have to decrease with age. Increasing each joints' range of motion helps protect against injury and increases your physical capabilities.

STRESS

All forms of exercise are terrific stress-management strategies. They provide us with excellent outlets for stress. Remember, we want to continually increase our potential outlets for stress. Exercise very nearly always works as a stress outlet. However, in addition to that I believe that it is important to practice some relaxation techniques or meditation exercises. Learning the relaxation response is just a matter of some effort and time. A variety of techniques are highly effective and readily learnable. These help you to relieve stress and keep you focused or centered in terms of your own personal life goals. These are not just beneficial from a psychological standpoint but beneficial from a physical standpoint as well.

Take good care of yourself physically and psychologically. This is one way that you are able to show affection or love for yourself. This is not selfish, evil, or anything else negative. When you take good care of yourself, you have so much more to offer others, especially those you love. Care for yourself so much that you take very good care of the only body that you will ever have. Your nutritional habits and exercise levels are among the most important things you can do to insure that your body keeps running smoothly for the long haul. Nutrition and exercise are so powerful that they can even postpone the emergence of difficulties that simply come from bad genes. Yes, good nutritional planning and appropriate, intelligent exercise can be extremely healthy behaviors to include in your life. However, some personal psychological principles are also crucial for the quality of life you are seeking. Of course, it is very important to establish some sense of meaning or purpose in life. Having a purposeful life is a basic human emotional need. This can be done through your work, through volunteer activities, or through a variety of other hobbies or leisure time activities. Remember, it is sometimes extremely helpful to find ourselves in the position to provide a service to others. We all can be significant. We all want to leave this world a better place than we found it. We can do this.

The importance of relationships cannot be overstated. Loving relationships are our emotional fuel. What food is to us physically, relationships are to us emotionally. We absolutely have to have them. Our personal happiness is highly dependent on the quality and, to some extent, the quantity of these relationships. Investing in the development and *maintenance* of close emotional relationships pays high dividends.

Hopefully I have demonstrated for you the vital relationship between changing our health behaviors and the emotional/psychological component. Separating them will never work very well. Health psychologists are constantly looking for better ways to help people engage in health enhancing behaviors while also helping them eliminate unhealthy behaviors (over-eating, stopping smoking, to name a couple)—a worthwhile endeavor, without a doubt.

Clinical and counseling psychologists often tend to focus more on mood disorders, anxiety disorders or other types of psychopathology in terms of prevention and treatment. Stress management and enhancing relationships are also part of their domain. Again, this is a critically important goal. In many ways health psychology and clinical psychology are two sides of the same coin, and together they can create a more profound "whole." Improving health and fitness levels can promote emotional health, and improved emotional functioning can increase the chance of success in terms of enhancing healthy behaviors, such as nutrition and exercise. Likewise, individuals contemplating any type of personal growth or physical fitness program need to remain aware of the connection of the physical and the emotional. This relationship is complex, and in some ways primitive and deeply ingrained. We cannot consistently, successfully deal with one without considering the other.

Meeting your emotional needs can charge up your attitude and make the self-improving lifestyle changes we have discussed very attainable. You can do this. You can make dramatic changes in your appearance, fitness, health and self-esteem. You can resurrect your physical abilities and your attitude. Remember, you are never too old to play or to laugh or to love. Do not give up on participating in life. It is much better to be on the playing field than it is to be in the bleachers just watching.

PUT IT ALL TOGETHER!

Okay, this is the best case I can make. I think your life is incredibly important, and I want you to maximize it. As I mentioned earlier, I think it is terribly important to watch the food that you eat and to try to stay with natural foods that form the primary menu for the human animal. Let's face it: we have learned much about nutrition, and it is time to apply that information to your life.

While we still don't know everything about exercise, we do know enough to appreciate how valuable it is in the enhancement of our lives and health. I think that it is incredibly important that you practice the three primary types of exercise. Exercise can transform your body, increase your health and is extremely valuable in the management of stress.

Stress management is always a work in progress. It is always an effort to keep in balance. Like life itself, it's an ongoing process. However, we know that it is very important to manage your stress in order to enhance your overall health, fitness, and happiness. Poorly managed stress is correlated with obesity, medical problems, and emotional difficulties. It is important to constantly try to expand your menu of activities that you feel passionate about. We desperately need things to look forward to, and we desperately need a reason to get up every morning.

Also, be mindful of the important people in your life. Never forget that loving relationships make life worthwhile and are important in attaining your happiness. Isolation nearly always yields hopelessness, depression, and disease. Try to fill your life with activities that make you feel good and are self-enhancing: not self-defeating. Seek out the company of people who make you feel good, invite you to be healthy, and shower you with affection.

Remember the interconnectedness of the mind and the body. All the tips that I have tried to give you to help you feel better emotionally will increase the chance that you can improve your nutritional status and your exercise level thus helping you to feel better physically. All the tips that I have tried to give you on improving your nutritional status and physical fitness can improve the way you feel emotionally. It is very helpful to focus some attention on both domains in order to maximize success. Remember, it can work either way and usually does.

Considering all the aspects of rejuvenation that we covered, we can evolve a prescription for health and happiness:

1. Eat sensible, "real" food. Avoid high glycemic carbohydrates, sweets, and fried food. Eat plenty of protein, low glycemic carbohydrates, and healthy fats.

2. Do the right kind of exercise: cardiovascular training, strength training (remember, everybody should lift weights), and flexibility training.

3. "Buff up" that self-esteem. Love yourself. Accept yourself. Practice becoming that person you want to be. Don't give up. Keep working at it.

4. Watch your self-statements. Decrease those negative self-statements and increase those positive ones. Pay attention to what's going on in your head.

5. Put your energies into your work. If you don't work, find engaging activities that you feel a passion for and focus on them.

6. Practice some type of relaxation training or technique. It's a small investment for a huge payoff. Stress is a killer.

7. Develop a full menu or repertoire of play activities and keep at it. Always be on the lookout for new ways to play.

8. Develop and maintain highly meaningful relationships—relationships where you love and feel loved in return. This is emotional "food." There is no happiness without this.

9. Structure your time. Stay busy with a sense of purpose.

10. Look for the opportunity to be of service to others. Remember, serving others is its own personal reward.

11. Embrace humor. Find a reason to laugh. Do it every day.

12. Practice forgiveness as a lifestyle. Remember, you reap what you sow. Oh yes, forgive yourself, too.

13. Don't make the mistake of over-interpreting your aging. The number is not important. How you feel is important. Don't use age as an excuse to throw in the towel on anything that brings pleasure and joy to your life.

A healthy mind makes it more likely to achieve a healthy body. A healthy body paves the way for a healthy mind. This is not a diet book. This is not an exercise book. My message here is the interconnectedness between the mind and the body. I want you to put it all together. Yep, the whole package. Okay, you can do this. You can really change your life. It takes some effort—sure. Nothing worthwhile is without effort. But, boy, is it worth it! You are worth it. Do it for you. Come on, in no time at all your birthday suit will fit you like a glove!

Abbreviated Table of Glycemic Index and Glycemic Load

REMEMBER, a GI less than 55 is considered low. A GI of 56–69 is considered medium. A GI of 70 or more is considered high. Also, a GL of less than 10 is low. A GL of 11–19 is medium. A GL of 20 or more is high. Although both Glycemic Indices are presented, I generally prefer the *glucose = 100 version.

Remember a serving size is generally about the amount of food that covers one quarter of a plate. Be sure to consider the Glycemic Load (the amount of carbohydrate present) as well as the Glycemic Index.

This is a developing area and all values must be assumed approximate. A GL indicated as —, means that value is not currently known.

Item	* GI (Glucose =100)	GI (Bread =100)	GL (per Serving)
BAKERY PRODUCTS **Cakes**			
Chocolate Cake, made from packet mix (Betty Crocker, General Mills, Inc.)	38 +/- 3	54	29
Sponge Cake, plain	46 +/- 6	66	17
Vanilla Cake, made from packet mix with vanilla frosting (Betty Crocker)	42 +/- 4	60	24
Muffins			
Apple, made with sugar	44 +/- 6	63	13
Apple, made without sugar	48 +/- 10	69	9
Bran (Grandma Martin's Muffins; Culinar Inc.)	60	85 +/- 8	15
Oatmeal, made from mix (Quaker Oats)	69	98 +/- 15	24
Pancakes, prepared from shake mix (Green's General Foods)	67 +/- 5	96	39
Waffles (Aunt Jemima; Quaker Oats)	76	109 +/- 6	10
BEVERAGES			
Coca Cola, soft drink	63	90	16
Apple Juice, unsweetened	40	57	—
Cranberry Juice Cocktail (Ocean Spray)	52 +/- 3	74	16
Orange Juice	46 +/- 4	66	—
Tomato Juice, Canned, no added sugar (Berri Ltd.)	38 +/- 4	54	4
Gatorade (Spring Valley Beverages Pty, Ltd.)	78 +/- 13	111	12
Powder Mix Drinks			
Quick, Chocolate, (Nestle), dissolved in water	53 +/- 5	76 +/- 8	4
Quick, Chocolate (Nestle), dissolved in 1.5% fat milk	41 +/- 4	59	5

Item	* GI (Glucose =100)	GI (Bread =100)	GL (per Serving)
BREADS			
Bagel, white, frozen (Lender's Bakery)	72	103 +/-5	25
Baguette, white, plain	95 +/- 15	136	15
Bread Stuffing, Paxo (Campbell Soup Co., Ltd.)	74	106 +/-10	16
Muesli Bread, made from packet mix in bread making machine (Con Agra Inc.)	54 +/- 6	77 +/- 9	7
Kaiser Rolls	73	104 +/- 5	12
Oat-Bran Bread – 50% Oat Bran	44	63 +/-10	8
Coarse, Rye-Kernel Bread, 80% intact kernels and 20% white-wheat flour	41	58 +/- 8	5
Rye-Kernel Bread, Pumpernickel	41	58	5
Coarse, Wheat-Kernel Bread, 80% intact kernels and 20% white-wheat flour	52	74 +/- 7	10
50% Cracked Wheat Kernel Bread	58	83 +/- 4	12
75% Cracked Wheat Kernel Bread	48	69 +/- 4	10
White Flour Bread	70	100	10
Wonder, Enriched White Bread	71 +/- 9	101 +/-13	—
Whole-meal Flour Bread	73	104	10
English Muffin Bread (Natural Ovens)	77 +/- 7	109 +/- 11	11
Healthy Choice Hearty 100% Whole Grain (Con Agra, Inc.)	62 +/- 6	89	9
Healthy Choice Hearty 7-Grain (Con Agra, Inc.)	55 +/- 6	79	8
100% Whole-grain Bread (Natural Ovens)	51 +/- 11	73+/- 15	7
Pita Bread, White	57	82 +/- 10	10
Wheat-flour Flat Bread	66 +/- 9	94	10

Item	* GI (Glucose =100)	GI (Bread =100)	GL (per Serving)
BREAKFAST CEREALS; RELATED PRODUCTS			
All-Bran (Kellogg's)	38	54	9
Bran Buds (Kellogg's, Inc.)	58	83 +/-11	7
Cheerios (General Mills, Inc.)	74	106 +/-9	15
Corn Chex (Nabisco Brands)	83	118 +/-11	21
Cornflakes (Kellogg's)	92	130	24
Corn Pops (Kellogg's)	80 +/-4	114	21
Crispix (Kellogg's Inc.)	87	124 +/-5	22
Froot Loops (Kellogg's Inc.)	69 +/- 9	98 +/- 13	18
Frosties, Sugar-coated Cornflakes (Kellogg's)	55	79	15
Golden Graham's (General Mills)	71	102 +/-12	18
Grapenuts (Kraft Foods, Inc.)	75 +/- 6	107 +/-8	16
Hot Cereal, apple and cinnamon (Con Agra, Inc.)	37 +/-6	53 +/- 8	8
Hot Cereal, unflavored (Con Agra, Inc.)	25 +/- 5	36 +/-7	5
Porridge	75	107	17
Quick Oats (Quaker Oats Co.)	65	93	—
One Minute Oats (Quaker Oats Co.)	66	94 +/- 10	—
Raisin Bran (Kellogg's)	61 +/-5	87 +/- 7	12
Rice Chex (Nabisco Brands, Ltd.)	89	127 +/- 5	23
Rice Krispies (Kellogg's)	82	118 +/- 6	22
Shredded Wheat (Nabisco Brands, Ltd.)	83	118 +/- 6	17
Special K (Kellogg's)	69 +/- 5	98 +/- 7	14
Total (General Mills, Inc.)	76	109 +/- 6	17
CEREAL GRAINS			
Barley	27	39 +/- 6	—
Buckwheat	49	70 +/- 6	—

Item	* GI (Glucose =100)	GI (Bread =100)	GL (per Serving)
Corn and Maize			
Sweet Corn, on the cob, boiled 20 min.	48	69	14
Sweet Corn	60	86	20
Couscous			
Couscous, boiled 5 min. (Near East Food Products Co.)	61	87 +/- 7	—
Rice, white			
Arborio, risotto rice, boiled (Sun Rice Brand, Rice Growers Co-op)	69 +/- 7	99	36
Long grain, white (Uncle Ben's)	56 +/- 7	80	24
Rice, long grain, quick-cooking varieties			
Long grain, white, precooked, microwaved 2 min. (Express Rice, plain, Uncle Ben's; King's Lynn)	52 +/- 5	74	19
Long grain and wild (Uncle Ben's, Effem Foods, Ltd.)	54	77 +/- 9	20
Rice, white high-amylose			
Brown, steamed	50	72	16
Instant rice, white, boiled 1 min.	46	65 +/- 5	19
Instant rice, white, cooked 6 min. (Trice Brand)	87	124	36
Parboiled rice	72	103	26
Converted, white, boiled 20-30 min. (Uncle Ben's, Masterfoods)	38	54	14
Converted, white, long grain, boiled 20-30 min. (Uncle Ben's)	50	72	18
Long grain, boiled 10 min.	61	887	22
Wheat			
Wheat, whole kernels	42	60 +/- 8	14
Bulgur wheat, boiled	46	66 +/- 4	—
COOKIES			
Oatmeal	54 +/- 4	77	9

Item	* GI (Glucose =100)	GI (Bread =100)	GL (per Serving)
CRACKERS			
Breton Wheat Crackers (Dare Foods, Ltd.)	67	96 +/- 4	10
Rye Crispbread	63	90	10
Stoned Wheat Thins (Christie Brown and Co.)	67	96 +/- 4	12
Premium Soda Crackers (Christie Brown and Co.)	74	106 +/- 5	12
DAIRY PRODUCTS AND ALTERNATIVES			
Ice cream NS (USA)	62	89	—
Ice cream, chocolate flavored	68 +/- 15	97	—
Milk, full-fat	40	57	—
Milk, skim	32 +/- 5	46	4
FRUIT AND FRUIT PRODUCTS			
Apple, Golden Delicious	39 +/- 3	56	6
Apple, NS	40	57	6
Apple Juice, unsweetened	40	57	12
Apricots, raw, NS	57	82 +/- 3	5
Apricots, dried	30 +/- 7	43	8
Banana, ripe, all yellow	51	73	13
Banana, slightly under-ripe, yellow with green sections	42	60	11
Cherries, raw, NS	22	32	3
Cranberry Juice Cocktail (Ocean Spray, Inc.)	68 +/- 3	97	24
Grapefruit, raw	25	36	3
Grapes, NS	43	62	7
Mango (*Mangifera indica*)	45	59	8
Oranges (Sunkist)	48	69 +/- 11	5
Orange Juice	46 +/- 6	66	12

Item	* GI (Glucose =100)	GI (Bread =100)	GL (per Serving)
Papaya	60	86	9
Peach, raw	28	40	4
Pear, raw, NS	33	47	4
Pear, Bartlett, raw	41	58 +/- 7	3
Pineapple, raw	57	73	8
Pineapple Juice, unsweetened (Dole Packaged Foods)	46	66 +/- 3	15
Plum, raw, NS	24	34	3
Prunes, pitted (Sunsweet Growers, Inc.)	29 +/- 4	41	10
Raisins	64 +/- 11	91	28
Strawberries, fresh, raw	40 +/- 7	57	1
Strawberry Jam	51 +/- 10	73 +/- 14	10
Tomato Juice, no added sugar (Berri Ltd.)	38 +/- 4	54	4
Watermelon, raw	72 +/- 13	103	4
LEGUMES AND NUTS			
Baked Beans, canned	40 +/- 3	57	—
Beans, dried, type NS	20	28 +/- 14	6
Black-eyed Beans	50	71 +/- 5	15
Butter Beans	36 +/- 4	51	7
Chickpeas	33	47 +/- 9	10
Haricot and Navy Beans, pressure cooked 25 min.	29	41 +/- 5	9
Haricot and Navy Beans, dried, boiled	30	43 +/- 5	9
Kidney Beans	23	33	6
Lentils, type NS	28	40	—
Lentils, red, dried, boiled	18	25	3
Peas, dried, boiled	22	32	2
Pinto Beans, dried, boiled	39	55 +/- 6	10

Item	* GI (Glucose =100)	GI (Bread =100)	GL (per Serving)
Worldwide Sport Nutrition Reduced-Carbohydrate Products (Worldwide Sport Nutritional Supplements, Inc.)			
Chewy Choc-Chip	30 +/- 4	43	4
Chocolate Deluxe	38 +/- 4	54	5
Peanut Butter	22 +/- 4	31	2
Strawberry Shortcake	43 +/- 4	61	6
NUTRITIONAL-SUPPORT PRODUCTS			
Choice, vanilla (Mead Johnson Nutritionals)	23 +/- 4	33	6
Ensure Pudding, old-fashioned vanilla (Abbott Laboratories, Inc.)	36 +/- 4	51	9
Glucerna, vanilla (Abbott Laboratories)	31 +/- 2	44	7
Resource Diabetic, French Vanilla (Novartis Nutrition Corp.)	34 +/- 3	49	8
PASTA AND NOODLES			
Capellini (Primo Foods, Ltd.)	45	64 +/- 8	20
Fettucine, egg (Mother Earth Fine Foods)	47 +/- 6	67	22
Instant Noodles (Mr. Noodle)	47	67 +/- 8	—
Macaroni, plain, boiled 5 min. (Lancia-Bravo Foods, Ltd.)	45	64 +/- 8	22
Macaroni, plain, boiled	48	69	23
Macaroni and Cheese, boxed (Kraft General Foods)	64	5	32
Rice Noodles, dried, boiled (Thai World)	61 +/- 6	87 +/- 9	23
Spaghetti			
Spaghetti, protein enriched, boiled 7 min. (Catelli Plus; Catelli Ltd.)	27	38 +/- 4	14
Spaghetti, white, boiled 5 min. (Lancia-Bravo Foods)	32	45 +/- 6	15

Item	* GI (Glucose =100)	GI (Bread =100)	GL (per Serving)
Spaghetti, white, boiled	33	47 +/- 9	16
White, durum wheat (Catelli Ltd.)	34	48 +/- 5	16
SNACK FOODS AND CONFECTIONERY			
Chocolate, milk (Dove; Mars Confectionery)	45 +/- 8	64	13
Chocolate, white (Milky Bar)	44 +/- 6	63	13
Corn Chips, plain, salted (Doritos original; Smith's Snack Food Co.)	72	103	18
Nacho chips (Old El Paso Foods Co.)	74	106 +/- 8	21
Roll-ups, fruit, leather-type snack	99 +/- 12	142 +/- 18	24
Kudos Whole-Grain Bars, chocolate chip (M&M/Mars)	62 +/- 8	89	20
M&M's Peanut (Mars Confectionery)	33 +/- 3	47	6
Mars Bar (M&M/Mars)	68 +/- 12	97	27
Peanuts	18	33 +/- 17	2
Popcorn, plain, cooked in microwave (Green's Foods)	55 +/- 7	79	6
Pop Tarts, double chocolate (Kellogg's)	70 +/- 2	100	24
Potato Crisps, plain, salted (Arnott's, Homebush)	57	81	10
Skittles (Mars Confectionery)	70 +/- 5	100	32
Snack bar, apple cinnamon (Con Agra, Inc.)	40 +/- 8	57 +/- 11	12
Snack bar, peanut butter and choc-chip (Con Agra, Inc.)	37 +/- 6	53 +/- 9	10
Snickers Bar (M&M/Mars)	68	97	23
Power Bar Sports Bar, chocolate	58 +/- 5	83 +/- 7	—
SOUPS			
Black Bean (Wil-Pack Foods, San Pedro)	64	92 +/- 9	17
Split Pea (Wil-Pack Foods)	60	86 +/- 12	16

Item	* GI (Glucose =100)	GI (Bread =100)	GL (per Serving)
Tomato Soup	38 +/- 9	54	6
VEGETABLES			
Green Peas, frozen, boiled	39	55	3
Sweet Corn, boiled	60	86	11
Carrots, NS	92 +/- 20	131	5
Potatoes			
Ontario, white, baked in skin	60	85 +/- 4	18
Russet, baked without fat	78	112	—
French Fries, frozen, reheated in microwave (Cavendish Farms)	75	107 +/- 6	22
New Potato	70 +/- 8	100	—
Sweet Potato	44	63	11
Taro, peeled, boiled	56 +/- 12	80	—
Yam	51 +/- 12	73	—

Meal Plans and Recipes

Jumpstart Stage

DAY 1

Breakfast:

> 2 slices of Turkey bacon
> Cheesy Omelet (page 221)

Mid-morning Snack:

> 1 oz. (approximately 16) pecan halves

Lunch:

> Chopped Tuna Salad (page 227)
> Small piece of fruit (from list on page 70)

Afternoon Snack:

> 1 or 2 Turkey Roll-ups (page 226)

Dinner:

> Grilled Salmon with Cucumber – Dill Relish (page 239)
> Sautéed Sugar Snap Peas
> Tossed salad

Dessert:

> Chocolate Crème Cup (page 246)

JUMPSTART STAGE
DAY 2

Breakfast:

> 4 slices of Canadian bacon
> Scrambled Eggs with Peppers and Onions (page 221)

Mid-morning Snack:

> 1 Mozzarella stick

Lunch:

> Grilled Salmon on Fresh Spinach Leaves—
> > use extra salmon from yesterday's dinner (page 229)
> Small piece of fruit (from list on page 70)

Afternoon Snack:

> 2 Celery sticks with 1 Tbs peanut butter

Dinner:

> 6 oz. Grilled chicken breast fillet
> Roasted Oven Veggies (page 240)
> Caesar Salad

Dessert:

> ½ cup fresh fruit cut up with 1 Tbs fat free whipped topping
> (optional)

JUMPSTART STAGE

DAY 3

Breakfast:

Chocolate Smoothie (page 225)

Mid-morning Snack:

1 or 2 Turkey and Cheese Roll-ups (page 226)

Lunch:

Chicken & Raspberry Salad (page 231)
Small piece of fruit (from list on page 70)

Afternoon Snack:

Cucumber slices with ¼ cup hummus

Dinner:

6 oz. Grilled beef fillet
Sautéed zucchini and squash with spray butter
Fresh spinach leaves with Warm Bacon Vinaigrette (page 233)

Dessert:

Peach Crème Cup (page 247)

JUMPSTART STAGE

DAY 4

Breakfast:

> 2 slices of Turkey bacon
> Veggie Frittata (page 224)

Mid-morning Snack:

> 1 Mozzarella stick

Lunch:

> Caesar Salad with Grilled Chicken (page 228)
> Sugar free Jell-o cup

Afternoon Snack:

> 1 small piece of fruit (from list on page 70)

Dinner:

> 6 oz Grilled Mahi Mahi
> Colorful Bean Salad (page 245)
> 1 fresh peach, sliced

Dessert:

> Lemon Lime Twist Cup (page 246)

JUMPSTART STAGE

DAY 5

Breakfast:

Turkey, Avocado & Cheese Omelet with Salsa (page 223)

Mid-morning Snack:

1 oz (approximately 24) whole cashews

Lunch:

"Everything but the kitchen sink" Salad (page 229)
Small piece of fruit (from list on page 70)

Afternoon Snack:

1 or 2 Turkey Roll-ups (page 226)

Dinner:

6 oz Pork Tenderloin
Stuffed Acorn Squash (page 241)
Fresh Green Beans

Dessert:

1 Sugar-free popsicle or fudgecicle

Jumpstart Stage

DAY 6

Breakfast:

    Fruit Smoothie (page 225)

Mid-morning Snack:

    Cucumber slices with ¼ cup hummus

Lunch:

    Crabmeat and Avocado Salad (page 227)
    Small piece of fruit (from list on page 70)

Afternoon Snack:

    1 oz or 45 shelled pistachios

Dinner:

    Marinated Balsamic Chicken (page 238)
    Stewed Tomatoes with Onions and Okra (page 242)
    Tossed dinner salad

Dessert:

    ½ cup fat-free, sugar free pudding

JUMPSTART STAGE
DAY 7

Breakfast:

4 slices of Canadian bacon
Scrambled Eggs with Peppers and Onions (page 221)

Mid-morning Snack:

2 Celery sticks with 1 Tbs peanut butter

Lunch:

Greek Salad with Chicken (page 230)
Small piece of fruit (from list on page 70)

Afternoon Snack:

1 Mozzarella stick

Dinner:

Beef and veggies on a skewer
Small Caesar Salad

Dessert:

½ cup Strawberries with 1 Tbs fat-free whipped topping
(optional)

JUMPSTART STAGE

DAY 8

Breakfast:

> 2 slices of Turkey bacon
> Turkey and Cheese omelet

Mid-morning Snack:

> 1 oz (approximately 12) walnut halves

Lunch:

> Mediterranean Salad (page 230)
> Small piece of fruit (from list on page 70)

Afternoon Snack:

> Veggies with ¼ cup hummus

Dinner:

> Grilled Tilapia with a Light Cream Sauce (page 239)
> Grilled Asparagus
> Roasted Confetti Peppers (page 244)

Dessert:

> ½ cup fresh fruit cut up with 1 Tbs fat free whipped topping
> (optional)

JUMPSTART STAGE
DAY 9

Breakfast:

    2 slices of Canadian bacon
    2 eggs over easy

Mid-morning Snack:

    1 or 2 Turkey wraps (page 226)

Lunch:

    Chicken Waldorf Salad (page 231)
    Small piece of fruit (from list on page 70)

Afternoon Snack:

    2 Celery sticks with 1 Tbs light cream cheese

Dinner:

    Stir Fry Chicken (cut chicken breast into strips, stir fry with
        1 Tbs of peanut oil and 1 Tbs lite soy sauce until done)
    Oriental Salad (page 243)

Dessert:

    Almond Crème Cup (page 247)

Jumpstart Stage

DAY 10

Breakfast:

> 2 slices of Turkey bacon
> Southwestern Omelet (page 222)

Mid-morning Snack:

> ¼ cup Hummus with raw veggies

Lunch:

> Chicken Caesar Wrap (page 232)
> Sugar-free Jell-o cup

Afternoon Snack:

> 1 piece of fruit (from list on page 70)

Dinner:

> Grilled Pork Chops
> Stuffed Butternut Squash (page 241)
> Black Beans

Dessert:

> Chocolate Crème Cup (page 246)

JUMPSTART STAGE
DAY 11

Breakfast:

    Chocolate Peanut Butter Smoothie (page 225)

Mid-morning Snack:

    1 Mozzarella stick

Lunch:

    Chopped Tuna Salad (page 227)
    Small piece of fruit (from list on page 70)

Afternoon Snack:

    1 or 2 Turkey wraps (page 226)

Dinner:

    Shrimp and Scallop skewers
    Oven Roasted Veggies (page 240)
    Small dinner salad

Dessert:

    ½ cup fresh fruit cut up with 1 Tbs fat free whipped topping (optional)

Jumpstart Stage

DAY 12

Breakfast:

>4 slices of Canadian bacon
>Veggie Omelet—your choice of vegetables

Mid-morning Snack:

>1 Mozzarella cheese stick

Lunch:

>Chicken and Raspberry Salad (page 231)
>Small piece of fruit (from list on page 70)

Afternoon Snack:

>1 oz (approximately 16) Pecan halves

Dinner:

>6 oz Grilled Grouper
>Sautéed Sugar Snap Peas
>Fresh Spinach leaves with Warm Bacon Vinaigrette (page 233)

Dessert:

>Strawberry Crème Cup (page 247)

JUMPSTART STAGE

DAY 13

Breakfast:

> 2 slices of Turkey bacon
> Cheesy Omelet (page 221)

Mid-morning Snack:

> 1 or 2 Ham and Cheese Wraps (page 226)

Lunch:

> Chef Salad with Turkey Breast (page 228)
> Small piece of fruit (from list on page 70)

Afternoon Snack:

> 2 Celery sticks with 1 Tbs peanut butter

Dinner:

> 6 oz Grilled Turkey Tenderloin filets
> Sautéed Zucchini and Squash
> Broiled Tomatoes (page 243)

Dessert:

> ½ cup fat-free, sugar-free pudding

Jumpstart Stage

DAY 14

Breakfast:

> 2 slices of Canadian bacon
> Turkey, Avocado and Cheese Omelet with Salsa (page 223)

Mid-morning Snack:

> 1 oz (approximately 31) Almonds

Lunch:

> Turkey BLT Wrap (page 232)
> Sugar-free Jell-o cup

Afternoon Snack:

> 1 small piece of fruit (from list on page 70)

Dinner:

> Orange Roughy with a Light Cream Sauce (page 239)
> Fresh Green Beans with Cranberries (page 244)
> Caesar Salad

Dessert:

> Lemon Lime Crème Cup (page 246)

Duration Stage
DAY 1

Breakfast:

¾ cup high protein cereal (such as Total Protein Cereal)
with ½ cup skim milk
½ cup of sliced strawberries

Mid-morning Snack:

1 oz (approximately 24) cashews

Lunch:

Chicken and Raspberry Spinach Salad (page 231)

Afternoon Snack:

1 small piece of fruit (from list on page 70 or 73)

Dinner:

Chicken breast marinated in Italian seasoning dressing
Colorful Bean Salad (page 245)
Small dinner salad

Dessert:

Chocolate Crème Cup (page 246)

Duration Stage

DAY 2

Breakfast:

> Southwestern Omelet (page 222)
> ½ cup of raspberries

Mid-morning Snack:

> 1 Mozzarella cheese stick

Lunch:

> Chicken Waldorf Salad (page 231)

Afternoon Snack:

> 1 –2 Turkey roll-ups (page 226)

Dinner:

> Grilled Pork Chops
> Stuffed Acorn Squash (page 241)
> Black Beans

Dessert:

> Almond Crème Cup (page 247)

Duration Stage
DAY 3

Breakfast:

Chocolate Peanut Butter Smoothie (page 225)

Mid-morning Snack:

Raw veggies with ½ cup of hummus

Lunch:

Tomato stuffed with tuna on bed of lettuce
1 cup of fresh fruit (from list on page 70 or 73)

Afternoon Snack:

1 oz of almonds (approximately 31)

Dinner:

Mahi Mahi with Avocado Mango Relish (page 236)
Grilled or sautéed Zucchini and Squash
Small dinner salad

Dessert:

1 cup of sugar-free, fat-free pudding

Duration Stage
DAY 4

Breakfast:

Veggie Frittata (page 224)

Mid-morning Snack:

1 piece of fruit (from list on page 70 or 73)

Lunch:

"Everything but the kitchen sink" Salad (page 229)

Afternoon Snack:

1 piece of reduced fat Provolone cheese and ½ cup of grapes

Dinner:

Stir-fry Chicken (cut chicken breast into strips, stir fry with
1 Tbs of peanut oil and 1 Tbs lite soy sauce until done)
Oriental Salad (page 243)

Dessert:

Lemon Lime Twist Crème Cup (page 246)

Duration Stage
DAY 5

Breakfast:

Turkey, Avocado and Cheese Omelet (page 223)

Mid-morning Snack:

1 oz (approximately 55) Pistachios

Lunch:

Greek Salad with Chicken (page 230)

Afternoon Snack:

1 small piece of fruit (from list on page 70 or 73)

Dinner:

Bacon Wrapped Sea Scallops (page 235)
Grilled Asparagus
Avocado Mango Tango Salad (page 242)

Dessert:

Fruity Crème Cup (page 247)

Duration Stage
DAY 6

Breakfast:

> 3 Eggs scrambled with 2 strips of lean bacon
> 1 slice of whole wheat bread toasted with spray butter

Mid-morning Snack:

> 1 small apple with 2 Tbs of regular peanut butter

Lunch:

> Chicken Caesar Wrap (page 232)

Afternoon Snack:

> 1 oz peanuts (approximately 61)

Dinner:

> Beef and veggies on a skewer
> Twice baked Sweet Potato (page 245)

Dessert:

> ½ cup mixed fruit with 1 Tbs of fat free whipped topping
> (optional)

Duration Stage

DAY 7

Breakfast:

¾ cup high protein cereal (such as Total Protein Cereal)
with ½ cup skim milk
½ cup of sliced bananas (slightly under ripe)

Mid-morning Snack:

8 baby carrot sticks with ¼ cup of fat free ranch dressing

Lunch:

Chopped Tuna Salad (page 227)

Afternoon Snack:

1 small piece of fruit (from list on page 70 or 73)

Dinner:

Grilled Tilapia with a Light Cream Sauce (page 239)
Sautéed Zucchini and Squash
Fresh Spinach leaves with Warm Bacon Vinaigrette Dressing
(page 233)

Dessert:

Chocolate Crème Cup (page 246)

DURATION STAGE

DAY 8

Breakfast:

Peach Fruit Smoothie (page 225)

Mid-morning Snack:

1–2 Turkey Roll-ups (page 226)

Lunch:

Chef Salad with Turkey breast (page 228)

Afternoon Snack:

1 small bunch of grapes with 1 slice of reduced fat provolone cheese

Dinner:

Grilled Salmon with Cucumber Dill Relish (page 239)
Sautéed Sugar Snap Peas
Marinated Cucumbers and Tomatoes in Italian dressing

Dessert:

½ cup sliced Cantaloupe with ½ cup reduced fat cottage cheese

DURATION STAGE

DAY 9

Breakfast:

> ½ cup Blueberries
> ½ cup old fashion Oatmeal mixed with ½ cup skim milk,
> 1 packet of sugar substitute and ¼ tsp. cinnamon cooked
> on low heat

Mid-morning Snack:

> 1 hard-boiled egg

Lunch:

> Grilled Salmon on Spinach Leaves—use extra salmon
> from yesterday's dinner (page 229)

Afternoon Snack:

> 1 piece of fruit (from list on page 70 or 73)

Dinner:

> 6-oz. Rib Eye Steak
> Roasted Confetti Peppers (page 244)
> ½ cup Black Beans

Dessert:

> Almond Crème Cup (page 247)

DURATION STAGE

DAY 10

Breakfast:

> ½ Grapefruit
> 3 Eggs, scrambled
> 1 slice whole grain toast with spray butter

Mid-morning Snack:

> 1 piece of fruit (from list on page 70 or 73)

Lunch:

> Turkey BLT Wrap (page 232)

Afternoon Snack:

> 2 cups light butter Popcorn

Dinner:

> "Rejuvenation Burger" (page 237)
> Small dinner salad

Dessert:

> ½ cup mixed fresh fruit

DURATION STAGE

DAY 11

Breakfast:

Strawberry Smoothie (page 225)

Mid-morning Snack:

1 pear with ½ cup reduced fat Cottage Cheese

Lunch:

Caesar Salad with Grilled Chicken (page 228)

Afternoon Snack:

Cucumber slices with ½ cup hummus

Dinner:

Shrimp and Scallops on a skewer
Oven Roasted Veggies (page 240)

Dessert:

½ cup sugar-free, fat-free pudding

Duration Stage

DAY 12

Breakfast:

½ cup Bananas (slightly ripe), sliced
½ cup old fashion Oatmeal mixed with ½ cup skim milk,
   1 packet of sugar substitute and ¼ tsp cinnamon cooked
   on low heat

Mid-morning Snack:

1 Apple with 2 Tbs of peanut butter

Lunch:

Turkey and Cheese wrap
½ cup of Grapes

Afternoon Snack:

1 oz (approximately 31) Almonds

Dinner:

6 oz Turkey Tenderloin filets
Colorful Bean Salad (page 245)
Broiled Tomato (page 243)

Dessert:

Fresh Strawberries cut up and mixed with 4 oz's of non-fat,
   sugar-free vanilla yogurt

DURATION STAGE

DAY 13

Breakfast:

Cheesy Omelet (page 221)
2 slices of Turkey bacon
½ Orange

Mid-morning Snack:

1 – 2 Turkey Cheese Roll-ups (page 226)

Lunch:

Mediterranean Salad (page 230)

Afternoon Snack:

1 part skim mozzarella stick

Dinner:

6-oz. Pork Tenderloin
Black Beans
Avocado Mango Tango Salad (page 242)

Dessert:

Chocolate Peanut Butter Crème Cup (page 248)

DURATION STAGE

DAY 14

Breakfast:

> 2 poached Eggs
> 2 slices of lean Bacon
> 1 slice of whole-wheat toast with spray butter

Mid-morning Snack:

> 1 piece of fruit (from list on page 70 or 73)

Lunch:

> Crabmeat and Avocado Salad (page 227)

Afternoon Snack:

> 8 baby Carrot sticks with ¼ cup of fat-free ranch dressing

Dinner:

> 6-oz. Beef Filet
> Stuffed Acorn Squash (page 241)
> Grilled Asparagus

Dessert:

> ½ cup Watermelon, cut up

REJUVENATION RECIPES

BREAKFAST

Cheesy Omelet

½ cup of egg substitute (or 2 eggs)
1 slice of reduced fat provolone cheese
Salt & pepper to taste

Lightly coat a medium skillet with cooking spray. Pour the egg substitute in the skillet. When partially set, place the cheese slice over the egg substitute and fold the omelet in half. Continue cooking until cooked through. Serve immediately.

Serves 1   Estimated Nutritional Facts

Per serving: 130 calories, 5g fat, 3g carbohydrates, 0 fiber, 19g protein
With whole eggs – 220 calories, 14g fat, 1g carbohydrate, 21g protein
(same for everything else)

Scrambled Eggs with Peppers and Onions

½ cup of egg substitute (or 2 eggs)
1 tablespoon chopped red bell pepper
1 tablespoon chopped purple onion
Salt & pepper to taste

Lightly coat a medium skillet with cooking spray. Sauté the peppers and onions until they are tender-crisp. Pour the egg substitute in the skillet. Scramble eggs until done. Serve immediately.

Serves 1   Estimated Nutritional Facts

Per serving: 130 calories, 5g fat, 3g carbohydrates, trace of fiber, 19g protein
With whole eggs – 220 calories, 14g fat, 1g carbohydrate, 21g protein
(same for everything else)

Southwestern Omelet

½ cup of egg substitute (or 2 eggs)
1 tablespoon chopped green bell pepper
1 tablespoon chopped yellow onion
3 tablespoons shredded reduced-fat Mexican cheese
2 tablespoons of salsa
Salt & pepper to taste

Lightly coat a medium skillet with cooking spray. In a small skillet sauté the peppers and onions until they are tender-crisp. Pour the egg substitute in the medium skillet. When partially set, add peppers and onions, then sprinkle cheese over egg mixture and fold the omelet in half. Continue cooking until cooked through. Spoon the salsa on top of omelet. Serve immediately.

Serves 1   Estimated Nutritional Facts

Per serving: 123 calories, 2g fat, 6g carbohydrates, trace of fiber, 20g protein
With whole eggs – 213 calories, 11g fat, 22g protein (same for everything else)

Turkey, Avocado & Cheese Omelet

1 cup of egg substitute (or 4 eggs)
2 slices of low-fat turkey breast lunchmeat, cut into bite-size
    pieces
2 slices of reduced fat provolone cheese, cut into bite-size
    pieces
1 Avocado, sliced
Salt & pepper to taste

Lightly coat a medium skillet with cooking spray. Pour the egg substitute in the skillet. When partially set, place the meat, avocado and cheese slice over the egg substitute and fold the omelet in half. Continue cooking until cooked through. Serve immediately.

Serves 2   Estimated Nutritional Facts

Per serving: 320 calories, 20g fat, 7g carbohydrates, 3g fiber, 25g protein
With whole eggs – 410 calories, 29g fat, 25g protein (same for everything else)

Veggie Frittata

½ cup of egg substitute
¼ cup of water
3 tablespoons nonfat dry milk
6 stalks fresh asparagus, cut into bite-size pieces
½ cup chopped yellow onion
¼ cup dry-packed sun-dried tomatoes
¼ cup sliced white mushrooms
1- tablespoon extra-virgin olive oil
Salt & pepper to taste

Boil 1" of water in a medium saucepan. Add the asparagus and cook, uncovered, until tender-crisp. Coat an ovenproof 8" skillet with cooking spray and place over medium-low heat until hot. Add the olive oil and sauté the onions and mushrooms until soft. Add the asparagus and sun-dried tomatoes, placing in a single layer covering the bottom of the skillet. Remove from heat.

Preheat the broiler. Mix together the egg substitute, water and dry milk. Pour over the vegetables. Cover and cook over medium-low heat for 6 minutes or until the bottom is set and the top is slightly wet. Place skillet under the broiler 4"–6" from the heat source until the top of the frittata is puffed and set, about 2 minutes. Be sure to watch it so that it does not burn. Serve immediately.

Serves 2   Estimated Nutritional Facts

Per serving: 111 calories, 1g fat, 20g Carbohydrates 5g Fiber, 10g protein

Protein Smoothie

> 1 – 2 scoops Whey or Soy Protein Powder Mix, any flavor
>   (use directions on container)
> 1 cup water*
> 6 to 8 Ice Cubes

Mix in blender until smooth, drink immediately to prevent settling.

* I prefer to use ½ cup water & ½ cup Milk Dairy Beverage for the additional protein (Hood Carb Countdown Dairy Beverage). You can also use skim milk.

Serves 1   Estimated Nutritional Facts

Per serving: 260 calories, 2g fat, 4g carbohydrates, 0g Fiber, 55g protein

Other Variations:

Chocolate Smoothie. Use chocolate flavor whey or soy protein powder, or 2 Tbs of Lite Chocolate Syrup (I prefer Walden Farms' Calorie Free Flavored Chocolate Syrup)

Chocolate Peanut Butter Smoothie. Same ingredients as above but add 1 tablespoon of regular Peanut Butter

Fruit Smoothie. Use vanilla whey or soy protein powder. Substitute half of your water for lite free plain yogurt and substitute your ice cubes for frozen strawberries, bananas or peaches.

**Nutritional information will vary and is not calculated.

SNACKS

Turkey Roll Ups

2 leaves of Romaine lettuce
2 slices of low-fat turkey breast lunchmeat
4 strips of red bell pepper
1 Tbs of Tangy Mayonnaise (see below)

Lightly spread the Tangy Mayonnaise on the lettuce leaf. Place lunchmeat on top. Add bell pepper strips and tightly roll up. You can also add a slice of low fat or fat free cheese.

Serves 1   Estimated Nutritional Facts

Per serving: 62 calories, 2g fat, 2g carbohydrates, trace of fiber, 12g protein

Tangy Mayonnaise

½ cup of fat-free mayonnaise
2 tablespoons of lime juice
1½ teaspoons of light soy sauce
1 teaspoon of minced garlic

Yields ½ cup   Estimated Nutritional Facts

Per tablespoon: 15 calories, 0g fat, 2g carbohydrates, 0g fiber 0g protein

LUNCH

Chopped Tuna Salad

1 cup chopped romaine lettuce
1 can (6 oz) water-packed tuna
¼ cup peeled, seeded & chopped cucumber
¼ cup chopped celery
¼ cup chopped tomato
½ cup chopped avocado
2 tablespoons Red Wine Vinaigrette (page 233)

Layer ingredients: lettuce, tuna, celery, cucumber, tomato and avocado. Pour 2 tablespoons of vinegar dressing over top. Serve immediately.

Serves 1   Estimated Nutritional Facts

Per serving: 379 calories, 17g fat, 13g carbohydrates, 3g fiber, 45g protein

Crabmeat and Avocado Salad

1 cup chopped romaine lettuce
1 can (6 oz) crabmeat, drained
½ avocado, sliced
2 tablespoons crumbled feta cheese
2 tablespoons Red Wine Vinaigrette (page 233)

Layer ingredients: lettuce, crabmeat, avocado and feta cheese. Pour vinegar dressing over top. Serve immediately.

Serves 1   Estimated Nutritional Facts

Per serving: 519 calories, 30g fat, 11g carbohydrates, 3g fiber, 46g protein

Chef Salad with Turkey Breast

2 cup chopped romaine lettuce
4 slices of turkey breast lunchmeat, chopped in bite size pieces
1 hard boiled egg, chopped
1 avocado, sliced
¼ cup crumbled blue cheese
4 tablespoons of imitation bacon bits

Equally layer ingredients onto two plates as listed: lettuce, turkey breast, avocado, blue cheese and bacon bits. Serve immediately with 2 Tbs prepared low-sugar salad dressing on each salad.

Serves 2   Estimated Nutritional Facts

Per serving: 356 calories, 27g fat, 13g carbohydrates, 5g Fiber, 24 protein

Caesar Salad with Grilled Chicken

1 cup chopped romaine lettuce
1 boneless, skinless cooked chicken breast, cut into strips
2 Tbs fresh grated Parmesan cheese

Layer ingredients: lettuce, chicken breast and Parmesan cheese. Serve immediately with 2 Tablespoons of prepared low sugar Caesar salad dressing.

Serves 1   Estimated Nutritional Facts

Per serving: 282 calories, 8g fat, 1g carbohydrate, 0g Fiber, 49g protein

"Everything but the Kitchen Sink" Salad

    2 cups chopped romaine lettuce
    1 small zucchini, sliced
    1 small yellow neck squash, sliced
    ½ cup sliced mushrooms
    ½ cup cauliflower and/or broccoli pieces
    ½ cup chopped cucumber

Layer ingredients: lettuce, zucchini, squash, mushrooms, cucumbers and cauliflower. Serve immediately with 2 Tbs of prepared low-sugar salad dressing.

**You may substitute any of the vegetables for others that is on the grocery list on page 71.

Serves 2   Estimated Nutritional Facts

Per serving: 80 calories, 1g fat, 15g carbohydrates, 4g fiber, 9g protein

Grilled Salmon on Spinach Leaves

    2 cups fresh spinach leaves
    1 (4 oz.) salmon fillet, ½" thick
    ¼ cup crumbled feta cheese
    2 Tbs Red Wine Vinaigrette (page 233)

Layer ingredients: lettuce, chicken breast and Parmesan cheese. Pour salad dressing over top. Serve immediately.

Serves 1   Estimated Nutritional Facts

Per serving: 425 calories, 30g fat, 4g carbohydrates, 0g fiber, 32g protein

Greek Salad with Chicken

4 leaves romaine lettuce, torn into bite size pieces
1 (4.9 oz portion) skinless, boneless cooked chicken breast,
    cut into strips
5 medium Greek olives, pitted
1 (4 oz.) roasted sweet red pepper (from a jar), sliced
¼ cup crumbled feta cheese

Layer the lettuce, chicken, olives, peppers and feta cheese.
Pour 2 tablespoons of prepared low sugar Greek dressing over top
and toss until evenly coated. Serve immediately.

Serves 1   Estimated Nutritional Facts

Per serving: 268 calories, 16g fat, 7g carbohydrates, 1g fiber, 45g protein

Mediterranean Salad (duration stage only)

4 leaves romaine lettuce, torn into bite size pieces
4 mini mozzarella balls, cut in half
1 (4 oz.) roasted sweet red pepper (from a jar),
    cut in to bit size pieces
3 quartered marinated artichoke hearts
5 medium Greek olives, pitted
2 tablespoons Red Wine Vinaigrette Dressing (page 233)

Layer the lettuce, mozzarella cheese, peppers, artichokes and
olives together. Pour vinaigrette dressing over top and toss until
evenly coated. Serve immediately.

Serves 1   Estimated Nutritional Facts

Per serving: 477 calories, 40g fat, 11g carbohydrates, 2g fiber, 28g protein

Chicken Waldorf Salad

    4 leaves romaine lettuce, torn into bite size pieces
    1 (4.9 oz portion) skinless, boneless cooked chicken breast,
        cut into strips
    6 seedless red grapes, sliced in half
    ¼ cup chopped apple with peel
    ¼ cup crumbled feta cheese
    10 pecan halves, chopped
    2 Tablespoons of Red Wine Vinaigrette Dressing (page 233)

Layer Ingredients: lettuce, chicken, apples and grapes. Top with feta cheese, pecans and dressing. Serve immediately.

Serves 1   Estimated Nutritional Facts

> Per serving: 553 calories, 23g fat, 14g carbohydrates, 3g fiber, 52g protein

Chicken & Raspberry Salad

    2 cups fresh spinach leaves
    1 (4.9 oz portion) skinless, boneless cooked chicken breast,
        cut into strips
    8 fresh raspberries
    2 Tbs slivered almonds
    5 small purple onion rings
    1 Tbs fresh grated Parmesan cheese
    2 Tbs Red Wine Vinaigrette Dressing (page 233)

Layer spinach leaves, chicken, onion rings, raspberries, almonds and cheese on a plate. Pour vinaigrette dressing over the top. Serve immediately.

Serves 1   Estimated Nutritional Facts

> Per serving: 469 calories, 24g fat, 13g carbohydrates, 3g fiber, 50g protein

Chicken Caesar Wrap

1 whole wheat tortilla**
1 (4.9 oz portion) skinless, boneless chicken breast,
    cut into strips
3 leaves of romaine lettuce cut into bit size pieces
1 Tbs fresh grated Parmesan cheese

Place chicken, lettuce and cheese in center of wrap. Add 2 tablespoons of any low carb, low sugar Caesar dressing. Roll up wrap and serve.

** Tumaro's Gourmet Tortillas is an excellent brand. However, if you cannot find it, any good low fat whole wheat (**not with enriched flour—see ingredients label**) will do.

Serves 1   Estimated Nutritional Facts

Per serving: 356 calories, 9g fat, 14g carbohydrates, 8g fiber, 52g protein

Turkey BLT Wrap

1 whole wheat tortilla**
1 slice turkey breast lunchmeat
2 slices bacon, cooked
1 leaf of romaine lettuce
3 thin slices of tomato
1 Tbs of Tangy Mayonnaise (page 226)

Spread mayonnaise over one side of the wrap. Then layer with lettuce, turkey, tomato and bacon. Roll up wrap and serve.

** Tumaro's Gourmet Tortillas is an excellent brand. However, if you cannot find it, any good low-fat whole wheat (**not with enriched flour—see ingredients label**) will do.

Serves 1   Estimated Nutritional Facts

Per serving: 245 calories, 11g fat, 18g carbohydrates, 8g fiber, 17g protein

---

SALAD DRESSING

Red Wine Vinaigrette Dressing

2 tablespoons extra virgin olive oil
4 tablespoons red wine vinegar
1 teaspoon Dijon mustard
2 Splenda packets

Mix all ingredients in salad croquet. Refrigerate unused portion.

Yields 3 Servings   Estimated Nutritional Facts

> 2 tablespoons per serving: 84 calories, 9g fat, 1g carbohydrate, 0g fiber, 0g protein

Warm Bacon Vinaigrette Dressing

4 slices of bacon, cooked and crumbled up
¼ cup apple cider vinegar
2 tablespoons extra virgin olive oil
1 teaspoon Dijon mustard
2 Splenda packets
Salt & pepper to taste

Heat in a microwavable measuring cup for 15 seconds or until warm. Pour immediately over Salad and serve.

Yields 4 Servings   Estimated Nutritional Facts

> 2 tablespoons per serving: 100 calories, 10g fat, less than 1g carbohydrate, 0g fiber, 0g protein

Oriental Dressing

¼ cup rice wine vinegar
1 Tbs lite soy sauce
2 Tbs Sesame oil
2 Splenda packets

Mix all ingredients in salad croquet. Refrigerate unused portion.

Yields 2 Servings   Estimated Nutritional Facts

2 tablespoons per serving: 70 calories, 7g fat, 2.5g carbohydrate, 0g fiber, less than a gram of protein

DINNERS

Bacon Wrapped Sea Scallops

20 large sea scallops
20 slices of cooked bacon
5 whole water chestnuts, diced
2 Tbs brown sugar
1 Tbs lite soy sauce
1 Tbs cornstarch
2 Tbs lemon juice
⅓ cup white cooking wine

Wrap each slice of bacon around each scallop. Skewer scallops then secure together with toothpicks. Grill scallops turning once. Cook until they are opaque in the center. In a small saucepan add chestnuts, brown sugar, soy sauce, cornstarch, lemon juice and white wine. Cook on medium low heat until sauce thickens, stirring occasionally. Place scallops on a plate, pouring the sauce over each scallop.

serves 4   Estimated Nutritional Facts

Per serving: 295 calories, 18g fat, 8g carbohydrates, 0g fiber, 17g protein

Mahi Mahi with Avocado Mango Relish
(Duration stage only)

2 - 4 oz Mahi Mahi
1 large avocado, chopped into cubes
1 mango, chopped into cubes
1/4 cup french white wine vinegar
1 package of Splenda

Flash freeze avocado and mango in freezer for 2 – 3 minutes before cutting into cubes. Place Avocado and Mango into a bowl and keep refrigerated until time to serve. Grill Mahi Mahi. Mix Vinegar and Splenda in with the avocado and mango. Lightly toss together. Spoon Avocado and Mango Mixture over Mahi Mahi and serve.

Serves 2   Estimated Nutritional Facts

Per serving: 403 calories, 17g fat, 40g carbohydrates, 12g fiber, 33g protein

"The Rejuvenation Burger"

1/2 lb ground sirloin
4 leaves of romaine lettuce
2 slices of Muenster cheese
2 slices of tomato
2 slices of purple onion
¼ tsp garlic powder
⅛ tsp onion powder
2 Tbs Dijon mustard
1 Tbs Worcestershire sauce
10 mild banana pepper rings, diced
1 Tbs of Tangy Mayonnaise (page 226)
Salt and pepper to taste

To make hamburger patties mix ground sirloin, garlic powder, onion powder, mustard, Worcestershire sauce, banana peppers, salt and pepper in a bowl. Shape into two equal patties. Cook over medium heat turning patties until they are thoroughly cooked. Remove from heat and place cheese slice on each patty. Divide Mayonnaise equally and spread over two of the lettuce leaves. Next place each hamburger patty on a lettuce leaf. Add Tomato and onion slice on top of each patty and top off with the remaining lettuce leaf. Serve with pickle spear.

Serves 2   Estimated Nutritional Facts

Per serving: 335 calories, 30g fat, 7g carbohydrates, 0g fiber, 53g protein

Marinated Balsamic Chicken

4 - 3.5 oz boneless, skinless chicken breast halves
½ cup balsamic vinegar
¼ cup red wine vinegar
3 garlic cloves, minced
1 tsp fresh oregano, finely chopped
1 tsp fresh thyme leaves, finely chopped
2 Tbs fresh basil, finely chopped
2 Tbs olive oil
2 Splenda packets
1 tsp salt
¼ tsp ground black pepper

Place chicken in a 9 x 13 inch glass casserole dish (plastic zip lock bag will also work). Put remaining ingredients into the blender or food processor and blend well. Pour vinegar mixture over chicken breast. Cover casserole dish with plastic wrap and refrigerate for 4 – 8 hours. Remove chicken from refrigerator and preheat grill. Discard vinegar mixture. Grill chicken 25 – 30 minutes or until fully cooked, turning several times during cooking.

Serves 4   Estimated Nutritional Facts

Per serving: 134 calories, 5g fat, 19g carbohydrates, 0.5g fiber, 23g protein

Grilled Tilapia with Light Cream Sauce

> 4 – 3.5 oz Tilapia
> 4 Tbs real (lite) butter
> ¼ cup white wine Worcestershire sauce
> ¼ cup fat free half & half
> ¼ cup dry sherry
> 1½ tsps. Paprika
> ⅛ tsp white ground pepper
> ¼ tsp salt

Preheat grill. In a small saucepan add butter. When butter melts, whisk in Worcestershire, sherry, paprika, pepper and salt. Meanwhile, cook fish 2 –3 minutes on each side. In saucepan add half & half and bring to a boil and then keep warm until fish is done. Place fish on plates and pour sauce over each fish.

*Also works well with Grouper and Orange Roughy.

Serves 4   Estimated Nutritional Facts

Per serving: 192 calories, 6g fat, 8g carbohydrates, 0g fiber, 20g protein

Grilled Salmon with Cucumber Dill Sauce

> 4 salmon fillets (4 oz each)
> ⅓ cup finely chopped cucumber, peeled and seeded
> ⅓ cup fat free sour cream
> ⅓ cup plain yogurt, lite
> 1 tsp fresh dill weed

Grill salmon. In medium bowl, mix together cucumber, sour cream, yogurt and dill weed. Refrigerate until time to serve. To serve, spoon the sauce evenly over each salmon fillet.

Serves 4   Estimated Nutritional Facts

Per serving: 241 calories, 16g fat, 2g carbohydrates, 0g fiber, 25g protein

SIDE DISHES

Oven Roasted Veggies

1 Zucchini, cut into bite-size pieces
1 Yellow neck squash, cut into bite-size pieces
1 medium red and orange bell pepper each,
    cut into bite size pieces
8 medium asparagus stalks, cut into bite-size pieces
1 small purple onion, cut into bite-size pieces
2 Tbs extra virgin olive oil
Salt and pepper to taste

Preheat oven to 450 degrees. Spray large baking sheet with cooking spray. Coat veggies with olive oil, salt and pepper. Place veggies in a single layer on baking sheet. Cook for 30 minutes or until tender and brown, stirring occasionally to prevent sticking.

Serves 4   Estimated Nutritional Facts

Per serving: 104 calories, 7g fat, 10g carbohydrates, 3g fiber, 11g protein

Stuffed Acorn Squash

1 medium acorn* squash, halved with seeds removed
1 small apple, diced with peel
2 Tbs real (light) butter
1 Tbs pecan pieces
1 package of Splenda
Salt and pepper to taste
2 Tbs fresh grated parmesan cheese

Preheat oven to 350 degrees. Place squash in a glass-baking dish cut side down. Add enough water to just cover the bottom of the dish. Microwave squash for 3-5 minutes or until tender. Drain water and turn squash over. Scoop out insides and place in a small bowl. Add apple, butter, pecan, Splenda, salt and pepper. Mix together and divide equal amounts of mixture into each shell. Sprinkle equal amounts of cheese over tops of both. Place squash in oven for 3-5 minutes or until cheese is melted. Serve immediately.

* You can substitute for butternut squash.

Serves 2   Estimated Nutritional Facts

Per serving: 196 calories, 10g fat, 26g carbohydrates, 4g fiber, 5g protein

Stewed Tomatoes with Onions and Okra

2 large tomatoes, peeled, seeded, and chopped
1 cup chopped onion
1 cup chopped green bell pepper
1 cup okra, sliced
1 clove garlic, minced
¼ tsp garlic powder
1 Tbs red wine vinegar
1 Splenda packet
Salt and pepper to taste

Spray nonstick skillet with cooking spray. Sauté onion, bell pepper and garlic until tender. Add tomatoes, okra, vinegar, salt and pepper to skillet. Once boiling, reduce heat, cover, and let simmer for 15 minutes stirring occasionally.

Serves 4   Estimated Nutritional Facts

Per serving: 54 calories, 0.5g fat, 12g carbohydrates, Less than 1g of fiber, 8g protein

Avocado Mango Tango Salad (Duration stage only)

1 large avocado, cubed
1 medium mango, cubed
¼ cup french white wine vinegar
1 Splenda packet

Flash freeze avocado and mango in freezer for 2-3 minutes before cutting into cubes. Mix together vinegar and Splenda. Place cut up avocado and mango in a serving bowl. Pour dressing mixture over it then keep refrigerated until time to serve. Serve chilled.

Serves 2   Estimated Nutritional Facts

Per serving: 185 calories, 15g fat, 40g carbohydrates, 12g fiber, 4g protein

Broiled Tomato

1 large tomato, sliced in half
2 Tbs fat free balsamic vinaigrette
1 Tbs pecan pieces
2 Tbs fresh grated Parmesan cheese

Place tomato halves cut side up on a broiler pan rack. Pour one tablespoon of balsamic vinaigrette over each tomato half. Divide pecan pieces equally on top of tomato halves. Sprinkle one tablespoon of cheese over each tomato. Broil tomatoes 5–7 minutes, watching carefully so that cheese does not burn.

Serves 2   Estimated Nutritional Facts

Per serving: 68 calories, 8g fat, 10g carbohydrates, 0.7g fiber, 7g protein

Oriental Salad

2 cups iceberg lettuce head, shredded
2 cups cabbage head, shredded
1 cup bean sprouts
1 medium carrot cut into julienne slices
1 zucchini cut into julienne slices
1 - 6 oz can of water chestnuts, sliced
2 Tbs Oriental Dressing (page 234)

Serves 4   Estimated Nutritional Facts

Per serving: 121 calories, 7g fat, 14g carbohydrates, 2g fiber, 3g protein

Roasted Confetti Peppers

    1 medium red bell pepper
    1 medium yellow bell pepper
    1 medium orange bell pepper
    1 medium green bell pepper
    1 Tbs olive oil
    Salt and pepper to taste

Cut peppers into bit size squares. Place peppers in a bowl with oil, salt and pepper mixing to coat well. Spread peppers on a broiler pan rack. Broil 7–10 minutes or until roasted.

Yields 2–3 servings   Estimated Nutritional Facts

Per serving: 124 calories, 7g fat, 31g carbohydrates, 10g fiber, 5g protein

Sautéed Green Beans with Cranberries

    1 lb fresh whole green beans, trimmed
    2 Tbs real light butter, salted
    2 Tbs slivered almonds
    1/3 cup dried cranberries
    1/4 cup feta cheese
    1 package of Splenda
    Salt and pepper to taste

Place beans in a medium pot with enough water to cover beans. Cook beans until tender but still crisp. Melt butter in skillet. Add almonds, Splenda, and cranberries and cook for 1 –2 minutes stirring occasionally. Sauté green beans in skillet with almonds and cranberries for a couple of minutes longer. Sprinkle feta cheese over top. Serve warm.

Yields 6–½ cup servings   Estimated Nutritional Facts

Per serving: 106 calories, 5g fat, 13g carbohydrates, 3g fiber, 4g protein

Twice Baked Sweet Potato

1 medium sweet potato
1 Tbs light real butter, salted
2 packets of Splenda
2 Tbs fresh grated Parmesan cheese
Salt and pepper to taste

Pierce potato with a fork several times. Place potato in the Oven at 400 degrees, cook for 1 hour. Let potato cool for 5 minutes. Slice potato in half and scoop out insides into a bowl. Add butter, Splenda, salt and pepper. Mash together and place equal amounts into the skins of the potato. Sprinkle with cheese. Place in the oven for 5 minutes or until cheese is melted.

Serves 2   Estimated Nutritional Facts

Per serving: 105 calories, 9g fat, 28g carbohydrates, 4g fiber, 7g protein

Colorful Bean Salad

1 – 15.5 oz can of black beans, drained and rinsed
1 – 15.5 oz can of great northern beans, drained and rinsed
½ cup chopped red bell pepper
½ cup chopped yellow bell pepper
½ cup chopped orange bell pepper
½ cup chopped purple onion
½ cup red wine vinegar
¼ cup olive oil
2 packets of Splenda

Mix together in a large bowl beans, pepper & onions. In a small bowl mix together remaining ingredients and pour over bean mixture. Serve chilled. Stir bean mixture before serving.

Yields 8–½ cup Servings   Estimated Nutritional Facts

Per serving: 164 calories, 8g fat, 18g carbohydrates, 7g fiber, 6g protein

---
DESSERTS

Chocolate Crème Cup

½ cup part skim ricotta cheese
1 Tbs of a calorie free, sugar free flavored chocolate syrup*

Mix all ingredients together in a dessert cup and serve chilled. You can make these ahead. It will keep in the refrigerator for a couple of days.

*I use Walden Farms brand chocolate syrup. You may substitute chocolate syrup for ½ tsp unsweetened cocoa and 1 Splenda packet. However, the nutritional facts will change.

Serves 1   Estimated Nutritional Facts

Per serving: 160 calories, 10g fat, 4g carbohydrates, 0g fiber, 14g protein

Lemon Lime Twist Cup

½ cup part skim ricotta cheese
¼ tsp lemon extract
¼ tsp grated lime zest
1 package of Splenda

Mix all ingredients together in a dessert cup and serve chilled. You can make these ahead. It will keep in the refrigerator for a couple of days.

Serves 1   Estimated Nutritional Facts

Per serving: 160 calories, 10g fat, 4g carbohydrates, 0g fiber, 14g protein

Almond Crème Cup

½ cup part skim ricotta cheese
¼ tsp almond extract
1 package of Splenda

Mix all ingredients together in a dessert cup and serve chilled. You can make these ahead. It will keep in the refrigerator for a couple of days.

Serves 1 Estimated Nutritional Facts

Per serving: 160 calories, 10g fat, 4g carbohydrates, 0g fiber, 14g protein

Peach Crème Cup

1 cup part skim ricotta cheese
1 small peach,* skinned and mashed

Mix ingredients together in a small dessert cup and serve chilled. You can make these ahead. It will keep in the refrigerator for a couple of days.

*You can also substitute the peach for 6–8 strawberries. The nutritional facts will vary from below.

Serves 2 Estimated Nutritional Facts

Per serving: 197 calories, 10g fat, 12g carbohydrates, 1g fiber, 15g protein

Chocolate Peanut Butter Crème Cup

½ cup part skim ricotta cheese
1 Tbs of a calorie free, sugar free flavored chocolate syrup*
1 Tbs of regular peanut butter

Mix all ingredients together in a small dessert cup and serve chilled. You can make these ahead. It will keep in the refrigerator for a couple of days.

* I like Walden Farms brand. You may also substitute chocolate syrup for ½ tsp unsweetened cocoa and 1 packet of Splenda.

Serves 1   Estimated Nutritional Facts

Per serving: 262 calories, 18g fat, 7.5g carbohydrates, 1g fiber, 18g protein

APPENDIX C

Optional Strength
Training Exercises

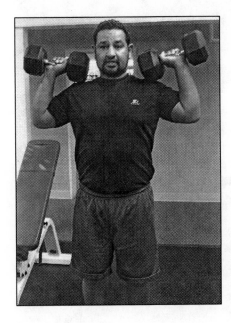

Dumbbell Press. With Dumbbells
at shoulder height, extend the left
arm fully. Then, while lowering the
left arm, raise the right arm. This is
one repetition.

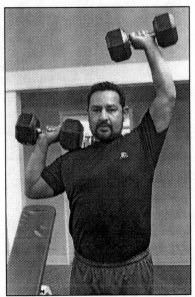

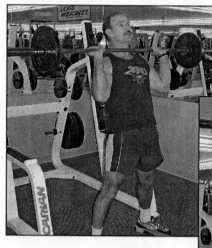

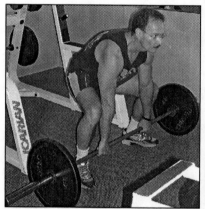

Barbell Press. With barbell at shoulder height, extend overhead, and then lower under control. This is one repetition.

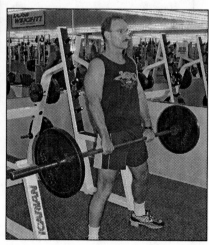

Dead Lift. With feet slightly wider than shoulders, bend and grasp the bar. Using predominantly your legs, lift to the standing position. This is one repetition.

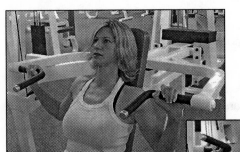

Machine Overhead Press.
Lift the weight up and return
under control. This is one
repetition.

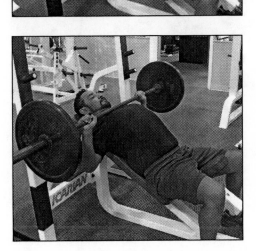

Incline Bench Press. This
is similar to the flat bench
press. This targets the
upper pectoral muscles. It
begins with the arms
extended. The weight is
lowered in a controlled
fashion to the chest and
then returns to the
extended position. This is
one repetition.

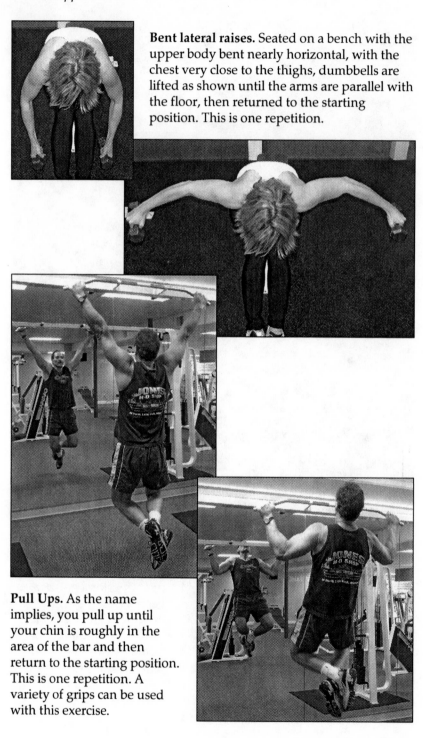

Bent lateral raises. Seated on a bench with the upper body bent nearly horizontal, with the chest very close to the thighs, dumbbells are lifted as shown until the arms are parallel with the floor, then returned to the starting position. This is one repetition.

Pull Ups. As the name implies, you pull up until your chin is roughly in the area of the bar and then return to the starting position. This is one repetition. A variety of grips can be used with this exercise.

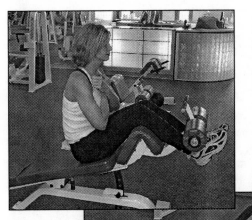

Slant Sit Ups. A slanting bench apparatus is used for this exercise. It can be adjusted to a variety of angles. The angles increase the amount of intensity on the abdominal muscles. It is a simple sit up where the intensity is high and repetitions stay fairly low.

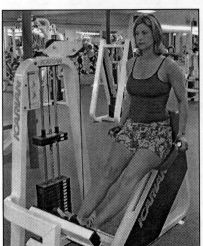
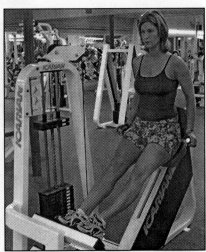

Calf raises. This is another machine for working the calves. The motion is begun with the heels low and then by tensing the calves the individual comes up on her toes. Returning to the beginning position is one repetition.

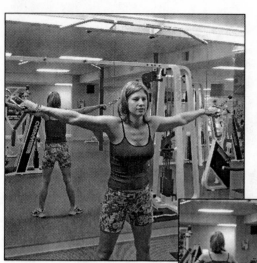

Cable cross over. If you have access to cables this is a good chest exercise. It can be done in a variety of ways and angles but basically you begin with arms extended and contract until the knuckles touch, as shown. Returning to the starting position is one repetition.

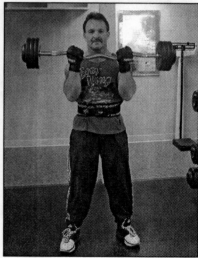

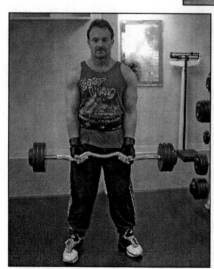

Barbell Curl. A variety of barbells are available for this type of exercise. Using the biceps the barbell is "curled" to shoulder height and then returned to the starting position. This is one repetition.

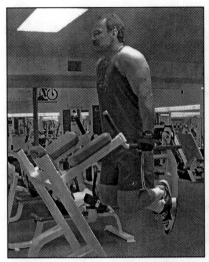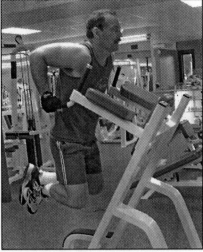

Dips. On a dip rack, begin with the arms in the straight, extended position. In a controlled manner lower your body until the upper arms are roughly parallel to the floor and then return to the starting position. This is one repetition.

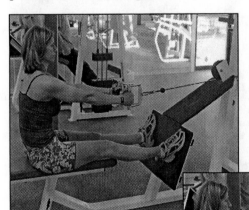

Seated Row. A variety of machines are available for this type of exercise. Begin with the arms in the straight position, and then pull in a rowing fashion with the resistance toward the chest. Returning to the starting position is one repetition.

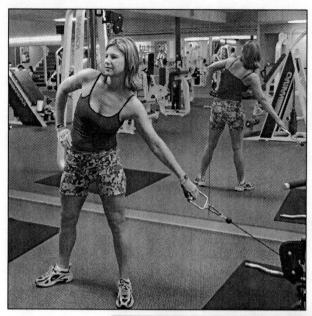

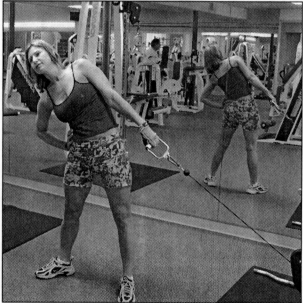

Side Bends. This can be done with the cable apparatus as shown or with a dumbbell. It is designed to work the obliques, or side of the torso. Using as large of a range of motion as possible move from one side to the other against resistance. When you return to the starting position, that is one repetition.

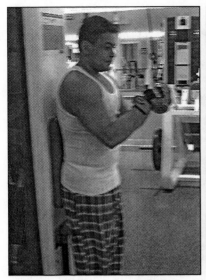
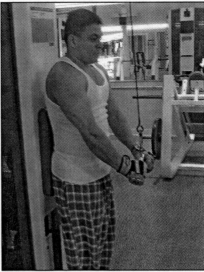

Triceps Push Down. A variety of grips or handles are available for this exercise. You begin as shown with the arms bent, and then, in a smooth motion, using the triceps, press straight down against the resistance. Once the arms are fully extended you return to the starting position. This is one repetition.

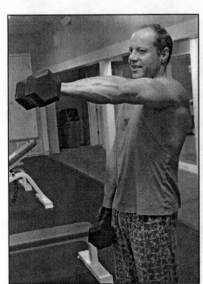
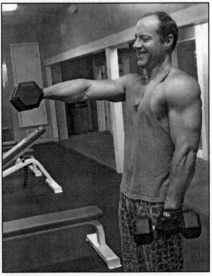

Dumbbell Front Raises. Begin with dumbbells in down position. Raise left dumbbell to shoulder level and stop. Return left dumbbell to starting position. Repeat with right dumbbell. This is one repetition.

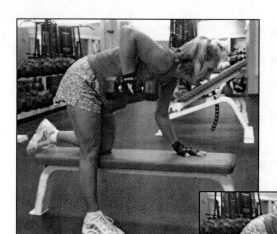

Dumbbell Row. Position on bench as shown, lift dumbbell to torso, then in a controlled fashion lower it. This is one repetition. Then repeat using other arm.

Dumbbell Flies. Begin with arms extended and dumbbells above your torso. Slowly lower dumbbells as shown. Keep the arms slightly bent for safety. Return to start position. This is one repetition.

About the Author

DR. KEN COUNTS IS A PRACTICING PSYCHOLOGIST in central Arkansas who attempts to integrate physical fitness aspects into his patients' treatment plans, when possible. This is because exercise has proven beneficial in terms of stress reduction, or stress management, and is often associated with improvement and self-esteem.

Ken Counts was a high school and collegiate athlete and has always been interested in physical conditioning. He received his Bachelor of Science degree from the University of Central Arkansas with a major in Psychology and a minor in Physical Education. After serving in the United States Navy in Vietnam, he returned to the same institution and completed the Master of Science degree in Psychology. Three years later he received his Ph.D. from the University of Southern Mississippi. This was followed by an internship at Central Louisiana State Hospital in Clinical Psychology. After he completed his training, he established his private practice and has practiced in central Arkansas since.

Dr. Counts has also continued to be an athlete—winning State, Regional and National Championships in Masters Power lifting and obtaining "All American" status in Masters Track and Field. Although a "senior," he continues to be active in these sports. He also encourages others to continue to be actively engaged in physical activity regardless of age. He believes that this is beneficial not only physically but also psychologically.

He was woven his interests in psychotherapy and physical fitness together in his clinical practice, whenever possible. He often approaches physical training as a psychologist and psychotherapy as a coach, injecting large doses of humor into both. He enthusiastically expects growth and improvement to evolve in both areas as they work together for the benefit of the whole person.

Dr. Counts continues to live and practice in central Arkansas.

Printed in the United States
73718LV00004B/109-117

9 781577 331575